AF342274

Clinical Record Book
for
Adult Health Nursing - II

Clinical Record Book
for
Adult Health Nursing - II

As per the Revised Nursing Syllabus

Dipak Sethi PhD

Dean and Professor
Noida International University
College of Nursing
Greater Noida, Uttar Pradesh, India

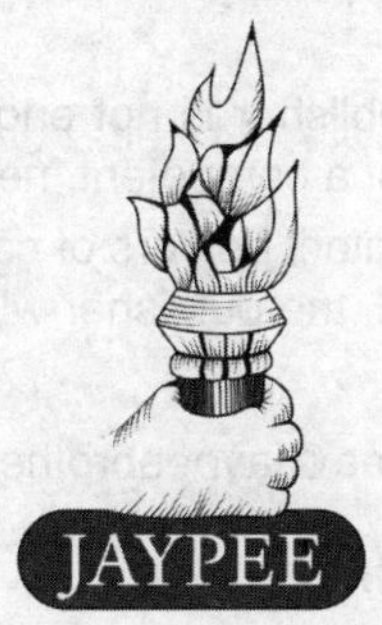

JAYPEE BROTHERS MEDICAL PUBLISHERS
The Health Sciences Publisher
New Delhi | London

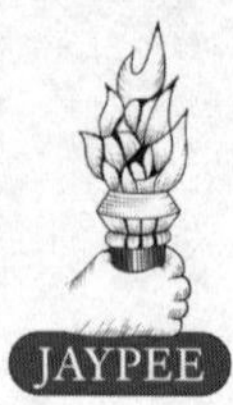
Jaypee Brothers Medical Publishers (P) Ltd

Headquarters

EMCA House
23/23-B, Ansari Road, Daryaganj
New Delhi 110 002, India
Landline: +91-11-23272143, +91-11-23272703
+91-11-23282021, +91-11-23245672
E-mail: jaypee@jaypeebrothers.com

Overseas Office

JP Medical Ltd.
83, Victoria Street, London
SW1H 0HW (UK)
Phone: +44-20 3170 8910
E-mail: info@jpmedpub.com

Corporate Office

Jaypee Brothers Medical Publishers (P) Ltd.
4838/24, Ansari Road, Daryaganj
New Delhi 110 002, India
Phone: +91-11-43574357
Fax: +91-11-43574314
E-mail: jaypee@jaypeebrothers.com

EU GPSR Authorised Representative

Logos Europe, 9 rue Nicolas Poussin
17000, La Rochelle, France
Phone: +33 (0) 6 67 93 73 78
E-mail: Contact@logoseurope.eu

Website: www.jaypeebrothers.com
Website: www.jaypeedigital.com

© 2024, Jaypee Brothers Medical Publishers

The views and opinions expressed in this book are solely those of the original contributor(s)/author(s) and do not necessarily represent those of editor(s) and publisher of the book.

All rights reserved. No part of this publication may be reproduced, stored or transmitted in any form or by any means, electronic, mechanical, photocopying, recording or otherwise, without the prior permission in writing of the publishers.

All brand names and product names used in this book are trade names, service marks, trademarks or registered trademarks of their respective owners. The publisher is not associated with any product or vendor mentioned in this book.

Medical knowledge and practice change constantly. This book is designed to provide accurate, authoritative information about the subject matter in question. However, readers are advised to check the most current information available on procedures included and check information from the manufacturer of each product to be administered, to verify the recommended dose, formula, method and duration of administration, adverse effects and contraindications. It is the responsibility of the practitioner to take all appropriate safety precautions. Neither the publisher nor the author(s)/editor(s) assume any liability for any injury and/or damage to persons or property arising from or related to use of material in this book.

This book is sold on the understanding that the publisher is not engaged in providing professional medical services. If such advice or services are required, the services of a competent medical professional should be sought.

Every effort has been made where necessary to contact holders of copyright to obtain permission to reproduce copyright material. If any have been inadvertently overlooked, the publisher will be pleased to make the necessary arrangements at the first opportunity.

Inquiries for bulk sales may be solicited at: jaypee@jaypeebrothers.com

Clinical Record Book for Adult Health Nursing - II

First Edition: **2024**

Revised Reprint: 2024, 2025, 2026

ISBN: 978-93-5696-959-9

Printed in India by K.K. Printers, Kundli, Haryana-131 028.

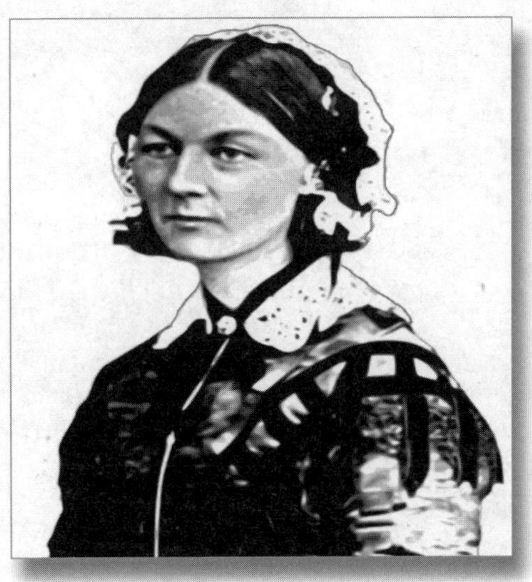

Pledge

I solemnly pledge in the presence of this assembly
To render nursing services with due respect
For the dignity and rights of the people I serve
I will, at all times, respect the values and beliefs
Of the people entrusted to my care
And will make no distinction of caste, creed or race
In the performance of my duties
I will strive in the practice of my profession
To promote health, prevent illness, alleviate sufferings,
And restore health of the people I serve
I will hold in trust personal information
Of a confidential nature
And use my best judgment in sharing this
With responsible persons
I will strive to maintain co-operative relationship
With fellow-workers in nursing and other fields
I will try to maintain standard of personal conduct
That will reflect credit upon my profession.
I will strive to observe the code of nursing ethics
As laid down by my profession.

Source: Nightingale Pledge and Code for Nurses 1973.

Preface

As the field of nursing education continues growing, the healthcare industry is constantly changing to acclimatize to the current needs of society. Similarly, nursing student's role is rapidly evolving as they are tasked with an even wider range of healthcare responsibilities given in their complex curriculum.

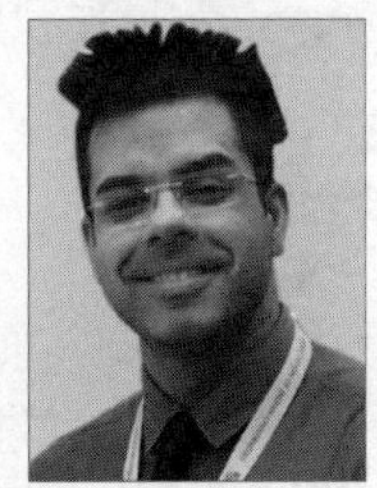

Clinical Record Book for Adult Health Nursing - II aims to help the nursing students to have handful of clinical requirements guide to facilitate them to complete clinical posting with effective utilization of given learning experience. It serves as a clinical guides for the students to understand comprehensive nursing care by gathering client information, performing nursing assessment and documenting nursing care provided.

In the word of uncertain strategies adopted by the different institutions of nursing, I feel this record book serves as a clear vision for the students to complete required nursing care plans, nursing case studies, case presentations, drug presentations, various reports, etc.

It is of utmost importance to the students to make their ideas clear in relation to the practice of nursing since they are going to care for the individuals, families, communities and their emotions. To fulfil this requirement, it is necessary to have common and well-approved strategies to follow in order to provide individual-based nursing care.

The development of this record book for BSc nursing 3rd semester resulted from the unexhausted effort committed to create excellence from most possible resources of national and international importance. Every effort has been made to present clinical formats with more practical orientation than theoretical outlook. The values and skills needed by the students in this era of dramatic changes in the healthcare delivery system, role of nursing in different settings have been given greater emphasis.

Comprehensive inclusion of clinical requirements is included to help the students to build their critical thinking skills and evaluate their own point of view. Every attempt is made to include total information for the students who can very well attempt to complete their clinical requirements successfully.

Dipak Sethi

Student Profile

Paste your passport size photo

Name of the Student: ....

PRN No.: ....

Batch: ....

Name of the Institute:..

____

Signature of Student

____

Signature of Subject In-Charge

____

Signature of Principal

Index

Nursing Management of Patients with ENT Disorders

- ☑ ENT Assessment
- ☑ Case Study
- ☑ Case Presentation

Nursing Management of
Patients with ENT Disorders

☑ ENT Assessment
☑ Case Study
☑ Case Presentation

Anatomical Diagrams of ENT

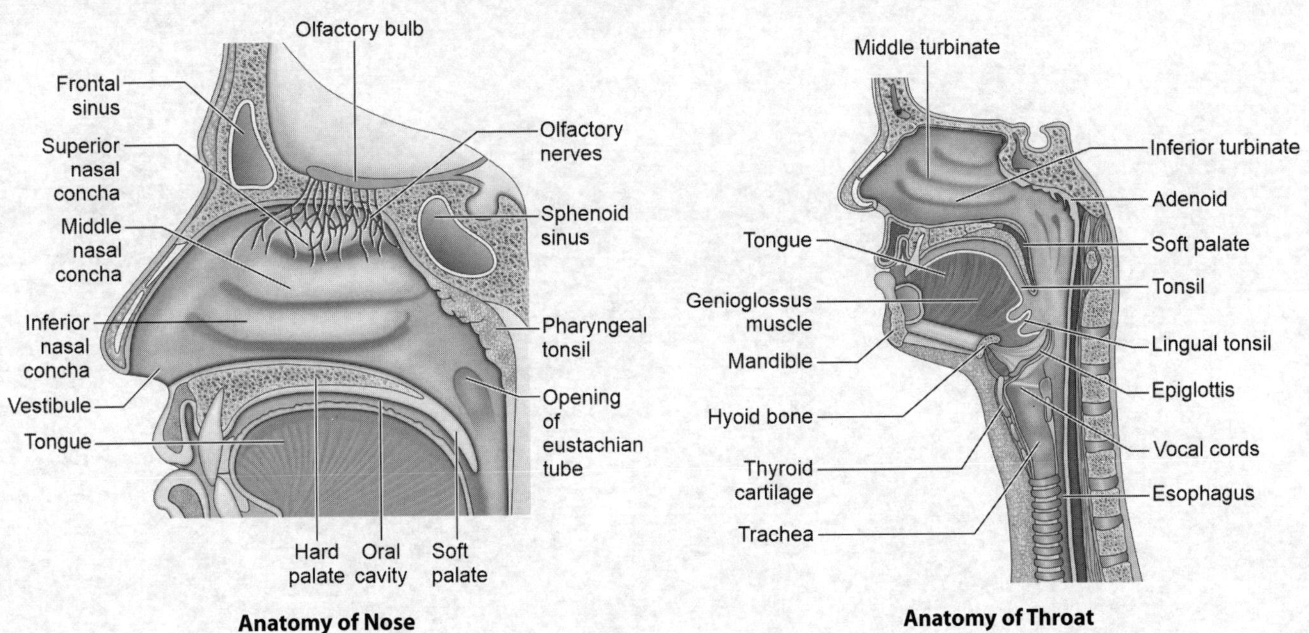

Anatomy of Nose

Anatomy of Throat

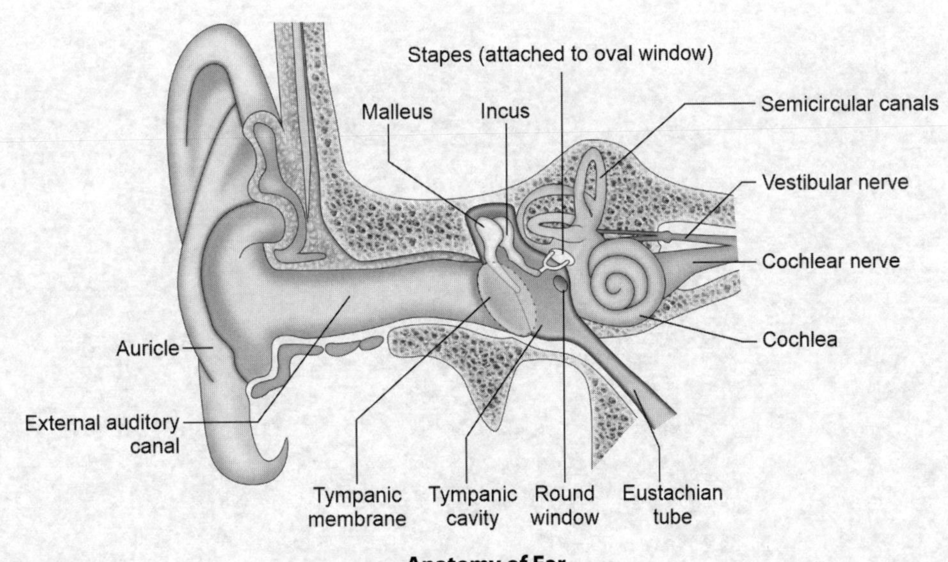

Anatomy of Ear

ENT Assessment

◼ EVALUATION CRITERIA FOR ENT ASSESSMENT

Maximum Marks: 25

S. No.	Contents	Maximum marks	Allotted marks
1.	Patient's history	02	
2.	Ear examination	05	
3.	Nose examination	05	
4.	Throat examination	05	
5.	Complication and prognosis	02	
6.	Health teaching	03	
7.	Conclusion	03	
	Total	**25**	

Remarks:

Signature of Student   **Signature of Supervisor**

Patient's Identification Data

- Name   :
- Age   :
- Sex   :
- Marital status   :
- Hospital registration no.   :
- Ward/bed no.   :
- Address   :
- Tel. no.   :
- Religion   :
- Education   :
- Date of admission   :
- Date of discharge   :
- Diagnosis   :
- Operation   :
- Date of operation   :
- Name of the doctor   :
- Occupation   :
- Monthly family income (₹)   :
- Nursing alert   :
- Sensitivity/allergy/precaution   :
- Weight   :
- Height   :

Informant

Information's relevant or not.

Chief Complaints with Duration

History of Present Illness

History of Past Surgical Illness: Illness/medications/any restrictions

Family History

S. No.	Name of family member	Age and sex	Relationship with patient	Occupation	Health status/ history of significant illness	Health habits

Family Tree

Socioeconomic History

- Occupation and social relationship:
- Monthly family income (₹):
- Health facility near home:
  - Type:
    - Hospital
    - Health center
    - Any other: If any other (specify)
  - Distance: __________ kms.
  - Transportation facility:
    - Yes
    - No
  - Housing: Type
    - Kutcha
    - Pucca
  - No. of rooms:
  - Toilet: Indian/western/temporary/open
  - Electricity: Yes/No
  - Drinking water source: Tap/well/pond/river/hand/pump

Dietary History

Health Habits: Functional Health Pattern

- Health perception/health management:

- Nutritional/metabolic:

- Elimination:

- Activity/exercise:

- Sleep/rest:

- Self-perception/self-concept:

- Role relationship:

- Sexuality/reproductive:

- Coping/stress–tolerance:

- Value/belief:

- Other comments/data:

Review of System

- **General:** The following characteristics of each symptom should be elicited and explored:

  - Onset (sudden or gradual):

  - Chronology:

  - Current situation (improving or deteriorating):

  - Location:

  - Radiation:

  - Quality:

  - Timing (frequency, duration):

  - Severity:

  - Precipitating and aggravating factors:

  - Relieving factors:

  - Associated symptoms:

  - Effects on daily activities:

  - Previous diagnosis of similar episodes:

  - Previous treatments:

  - Efficacy of previous treatments:

- **Ears:**

  - Recent changes in hearing:

  - Compliance with and effectiveness of hearing aid:

  - Itching:

  - Earache:

  - Discharge:

  - Tinnitus:

  - Vertigo:

  - Ear trauma:

  - Cotton swab use:

- **Nose and sinuses:**

    - Rhinorrhea:

    - Epistaxis:

    - Obstruction of airflow:

    - Sinus pain and localized headache:

    - Itching:

    - Anosmia:

    - Nasal trauma:

    - Sneezing:

    - Watery eyes:

- **Mouth and throat:**

    - Hoarseness or recent voice change:

    - Dental status:

    - Oral lesions:

    - Bleeding gums:

    - Sore throat:

    - Dysphagia:

- **Neck:**

    - Pain:

    - Swelling:

    - Enlarged glands:

    - Increasing headache associated with flexing of the neck:

- **Medical history (general):**

    - Medical conditions and surgeries:

    - Allergies (seasonal as well as others):

    - Medication currently used (prescription, oral contraceptives, over the counter):

- **Medical history (specific to ENT):**

  - Frequent ear or throat infections:

  - Sinusitis:

  - Trauma to the head or ENT area:

  - ENT surgery:

  - Hearing loss or audiometric screening results indicating hearing loss:

  - Seasonal allergies:

  - Asthma:

  - Chronic cough:

  - Meniere's disease:

  - ENT cancer:

- **Personal and social history (specific to ENT):**

  - Others at home with similar symptoms:

  - Smoking:

  - Alcohol use:

  - Exposure to mould:

  - Frequent immersion of ears in water (e.g., swimming, bathing):

  - Use of foreign object to clean ear:

  - Use of ear protection:

  - Crowded living conditions:

  - Sexual activity:

  - Personal and dental hygiene habits:

  - Exposure to cigarette smoke, wood smoke or other respiratory irritants:

  - Recent air travel or scuba diving:

  - Occupational exposure to toxins or loud noises:

PHYSICAL ASSESSMENT OF THE EARS, NOSE AND THROAT

- **Vitals:**

  - Temperature:

  - Pulse:

  - Respiration:

  - SpO_2:

  - Blood pressure (BP):

- **General appearance:**

  - Apparent state of health:

  - Appearance of comfort or distress:

  - Color:

  - Nutritional status:

  - State of hydration:

  - Hygiene:

  - Match between appearance and stated age:

  - Difficulty with gait or balance:

  - Piercings and tattoos:

- **Ears inspection:**

  - Pinna:

    - Lesions:

    - Abnormal appearance or position:

    - Look at the skin covering the mastoid process:

    - Behind pinna for redness or swelling:

    - Gently pull the pinna forward:

–   Canal (discharge, swelling, redness, wax, foreign bodies):

–   Tympanic membrane: Color, light reflex, landmarks, bulging or retraction, perforation, scarring, air bubbles, fluid level:

–   Estimate hearing with watch or whisper test:

–   If whisper test fails, perform Weber and Rinne tests with a 512-hertz tuning fork palpation:

–   Tenderness over tragus or on manipulation of the pinna:

–   Tenderness on tapping of mastoid process:

–   Size and tenderness of pre, post auricular and occipital nodes:

- **Nose and sinuses:**

  –   Inspection:

  - External (inflammation, deformity, discharge or bleeding):

  - Internal (color of mucosa, edema, deviated or perforated septum, polyps, bleeding):

  - Observe nasal versus mouth breathing:

  –   Palpation:

  - Sinus and nasal tenderness:

  –   Percussion:

  - Sinus and nasal tenderness:

- **Mouth and throat:**

  –   Inspection:

  - Lips (color, lesions, symmetry):

  - Oral cavity (breath odor, color, lesions of buccal mucosa):

  - Teeth and gums (redness, swelling, caries, bleeding):

  - Tongue: Color, texture, lesions, tenderness of floor of mouth:

  - Throat and pharynx (color, exudates, uvula, tonsillar symmetry and enlargement, masses):

- **Neck:**

    - Inspection:

        ◆ Symmetry:

        ◆ Swelling:

        ◆ Masses:

        ◆ Active range of motion:

        ◆ Thyroid enlargement:

- **Palpation:**

    - Tenderness, enlargement, mobility, contour and consistency of nodes and masses:

    - Thyroid (size, consistency, contour, position, tenderness):

    - Parotid:

Other Investigations

Date	Investigations done	Normal value	Patient value	Inference

Drug Study

S. No.	Drug trade name	Pharmacological name	Dose and frequency	Route	Action	Side effects and drug interaction	Nurses responsibility

Complications and Prognosis

Health Teaching

Summary and Conclusion

Bibliography

Case Study

■ EVALUATION CRITERIA FOR NURSING CASE STUDY

Maximum Marks: 100

S. No.	Contents	Maximum marks	Marks obtained
1.	Patient's history	04	
2.	Physical examination	04	
3.	Anatomy and physiology	05	
4.	Incidence and etiology	05	
5.	Pathophysiology	05	
6.	Clinical manifestations	06	
7.	Investigations	04	
8.	Complication and prognosis	05	
9.	Management: Medical and surgical	12	
10.	Drug study	10	
11.	Nursing care plan	15	
12.	Nurses' notes	08	
13.	Health education	06	
14.	Discharge planning	05	
15.	Conclusion and research evidence	03	
16.	Bibliography	03	
	Total	**100**	

Remarks:

Signature of Student   **Signature of Supervisor**

PROFORMA AND GUIDELINE FOR NURSING CASE STUDY

Introduction

Purposes of the Study

Objectives of the Study

Duration of the Study

Patient's Identification Data

- Name :
- Age :
- Sex :
- Marital status :
- Hospital registration no. :
- Ward/bed no. :
- Address :
- Tel. no. :
- Religion :
- Education :
- Date of admission :
- Date of discharge :
- Diagnosis :
- Operation :
- Date of operation :
- Name of the doctor :
- Occupation :
- Monthly family income (₹) :
- Nursing alert :
- Sensitivity/allergy/precaution :
- Weight :
- Height :

Informant

Information's relevant or not.

Chief Complaints with Duration

History of Present Illness

History of Past Medical Illness: Illness/medications/any restrictions.

History of Past Surgical Illness: Illness/medications/any restrictions.

Obstetrical History

Family History

S. No.	Name of family member	Age and sex	Relationship with patient	Occupation	Health status/ history of significant illness	Health habits

Family Tree

Socioeconomic History

- Occupation and social relationship:
- Monthly family income (₹):
- Health facility near home:
    - Type:
        - Hospital
        - Health center
        - Any other: If any other (specify)
    - Distance: _________ kms.
    - Transportation facility:
        - Yes
        - No
    - Housing: Type
        - Kutcha
        - Pucca
    - No. of rooms:
    - Toilet: Indian/western/temporary/open
    - Electricity: Yes/No
    - Drinking water source: Tap/well/pond/river/hand/pump

Dietary History

Health Habits: Functional Health Pattern

- Health perception/health management:

- Nutritional/metabolic:

- Elimination:

- Activity/exercise:

- Sleep/rest:

- Self-perception/self-concept:

- Role relationship:

- Sexuality/reproductive:

- Coping/stress–tolerance:

- Value/belief:

- Other comments/data:

Physical Examination

General Appearance

Height

Weight

Vital Signs

S. No.	Vital sign	Patient value	Normal value	Remarks
1.	Temperature			
2.	Pulse			
3.	Respiration			
4.	Blood pressure			

Head

- Scalp:
- Face:
- Sinus:
- Nodes:

Eyes

- Ocular movement:
- Pupils:
- Sclera:
- Cornea:

Ears

- External structures:
- Hearing:

Nose

- External structure:
- Septum:
- Mucous membrane:
- Patency:
- Olfactory sense:

Mouth

- Buccal mucosa:
- Gums:
- Teeth:
- Palates and uvula:
- Tonsillar area:
- Voice breath:

Neck

- Muscles:
- Trachea:
- Thyroid:
- Nodes:
- Vein distension:

Thorax

- Chest shape:
- Respiratory rate:
- Type of respiration:
- Thoracic expansion:
- Palpation:
- Percussion:
- Breath sounds:

Cardiovascular System

- Precordium: Inspection:
- Palpation:
- Auscultation:
- Apical rate and rhythm:

Central and Peripheral Vessels

- Carotid arteries:
- Peripheral pulses—Brachial:
- Radial:
- Femoral:
- Popliteal:
- Dorsal pedal:

- Posterior tibial:

- Capillary refill:

Abdomen

- Inspection:

- Auscultation:

- Percussion:

- Palpation:

Musculoskeletal System

- Gait:

- Upper extremities:

- Lower extremities:

- Muscle strength:

- Joints:

- Range of motion:

- Spine:

Nervous System

- Mental status:

  - Language:

  - Orientation:

  - Memory attention span:

- Level of consciousness (GCS):

- Cranial nerves:

- Deep tendon reflex:

- Gross and fine motor function of UE and LE:

- Sensory function:

  - Light touch:

  - Pain:

  - Temperature:

- Position:

Genitalia and Rectal Examination

- Inspection:

- Palpation:

Comparison of the Patient's Disease with Book Picture

- Definition

- Anatomy and physiology

- Incidence

- Etiology

Book picture	Patient picture

- Pathophysiology

- Signs and symptoms

- Diagnosis provisional and final

Book picture	Patient picture

Investigations

Date	Investigations done	Normal value	Patient value	Inference

Management: Medical or Surgical

Drug Study

S. No.	Drug trade name	Pharmacological name	Dose and frequency	Route	Action	Side effects and drug interaction	Nurses responsibility

Nursing Care Plan

Nursing assessment: Subjective and objective data	Nursing diagnosis	Goals	Nursing intervention		Rationale	Evaluation
			Planned	Implemented		

Nurses' Notes

Time	Medication	Diet/nutrition	Observation/intervention/evaluation	Signature

Complications and Prognosis

Health Teaching

Discharge Planning/Notes

Summary and Conclusion

Bibliography

Case Presentation

■ EVALUATION CRITERIA FOR NURSING CASE PRESENTATION

Maximum Marks: 100

S. No.	Contents	Maximum marks	Marks obtained
1.	Assessment	10	
2.	Co-relation with patient and book	15	
3.	Drug study	06	
4.	Nursing care plan	25	
5.	Nurses' notes	05	
6.	Health education	06	
7.	Use of AV Aids	08	
8.	Physical arrangement	05	
9.	Group participation	10	
10.	Effectiveness of presentation	05	
11.	Bibliography	05	
	Total	**100**	

Remarks:

Signature of Student　　　　　　　　　　　　　　　　**Signature of Supervisor**

PROFORMA AND GUIDELINE FOR NURSING CASE PRESENTATION

Patient's Identification Data

- Name   :
- Age   :
- Sex   :
- Marital status   :
- Hospital registration no.   :
- Ward/bed no.   :
- Address   :
- Tel. no.   :
- Religion   :
- Education   :
- Date of admission   :
- Date of discharge   :
- Diagnosis   :
- Operation   :
- Date of operation   :
- Name of the doctor   :
- Occupation   :
- Monthly family income (₹)   :
- Nursing alert   :
- Sensitivity/allergy/precaution   :
- Weight   :
- Height   :

Informant

Information's relevant or not.

Chief Complaints with Duration

History of Present Illness

History of Past Medical Illness: Illness/medications/any restrictions.

History of Past Surgical Illness: Illness/medications/any restrictions.

Obstetrical History

Family History

S. No.	Name of family member	Age and sex	Relationship with patient	Occupation	Health status/ history of significant illness	Health habits

Family Tree

Socioeconomic History

- Occupation and social relationship:
- Monthly family income (₹):
- Health facility near home:
  - Type:
    - Hospital
    - Health center
    - Any other: If any other (specify)
  - Distance: __________ kms.
  - Transportation facility:
    - Yes
    - No
  - Housing: Type
    - Kutcha
    - Pucca
  - No. of rooms:
  - Toilet: Indian/western/temporary/open
  - Electricity: Yes/No
  - Drinking water source: Tap/well/pond/river/hand/pump

Dietary History

Health Habits: Functional Health Pattern

- Health perception/health management:

- Nutritional/metabolic:

- Elimination:

- Activity/exercise:

- Sleep/rest:

- Self-perception/self-concept:

- Role relationship:

- Sexuality/reproductive:

- Coping/stress–tolerance:

- Value/belief:

- Other comments/data:

Physical Examination

General Appearance

Height

Weight

Vital Signs

S. No.	Vital sign	Patient value	Normal value	Remarks
1.	Temperature			
2.	Pulse			
3.	Respiration			
4.	Blood pressure			

Head

- Scalp:
- Face:
- Sinus:
- Nodes:

Eyes

- Ocular movement:
- Pupils:
- Sclera:
- Cornea:

Ears

- External structures:
- Hearing:

Nose

- External structure:
- Septum:
- Mucous membrane:
- Patency:
- Olfactory sense:

Mouth

- Buccal mucosa:

- Gums:

- Teeth:

- Palates and uvula:

- Tonsillar area:

- Voice breath:

Neck

- Muscles:

- Trachea:

- Thyroid:

- Nodes:

- Vein distension:

Thorax

- Chest shape:

- Respiratory rate:

- Type of respiration:

- Thoracic expansion:

- Palpation:

- Percussion:

- Breath sounds:

Cardiovascular System

- Precordium—Inspection:

- Palpation:

- Auscultation:

- Apical rate and rhythm:

Central and Peripheral Vessels

- Carotid arteries:

- Peripheral pulses—Brachial:

- Radial:

- Femoral:
- Popliteal:
- Dorsal pedal:
- Posterior tibial:
- Capillary refill:

Abdomen

- Inspection:
- Auscultation:
- Percussion:
- Palpation:

Musculoskeletal System

- Gait:
- Upper extremities:
- Lower extremities:
- Muscle strength:
- Joints:
- Range of motion:
- Spine:

Nervous System

- Mental status:
    - Language:
    - Orientation:
    - Memory attention span:
- Level of consciousness (GCS):
- Cranial nerves:
- Deep tendon reflex:
- Gross and fine motor function of UE and LE:
- Sensory function:
    - Light touch:
    - Pain:
    - Temperature:
- Position:

Genitalia and Rectal Examination

- Inspection:

- Palpation:

Comparison of the Patient's Disease with Book Picture

- Anatomy and physiology

- Incidence

- Etiology

Book picture	Patient picture

- Pathophysiology

- Clinical manifestations

Book picture	Patient picture

- Diagnosis provisional and final

Book picture	Patient picture

Investigations

Date	Investigations done	Normal value	Patient value	Inference

Management: Medical or Surgical

Drug Study

S. No.	Drug trade name	Pharmacological name	Dose and frequency	Route	Action	Side effects and drug interaction	Nurses responsibility

Nursing Care Plan

Nursing assessment: Subjective and objective data	Nursing diagnosis	Goals	Nursing intervention		Rationale	Evaluation
			Planned	Implemented		

Nurses' Notes

Time	Medication	Diet/nutrition	Observation/intervention/evaluation	Signature

Complications and Prognosis

Health Teaching

Discharge Planning/Notes

Summary and Conclusion

**Bibliography

Nursing Management of Patients with Eye Disorders

- ☑ Eye Assessment
- ☑ Case Study
- ☑ Case Presentation
- ☑ Health Teaching

Anatomical Diagrams of Eye

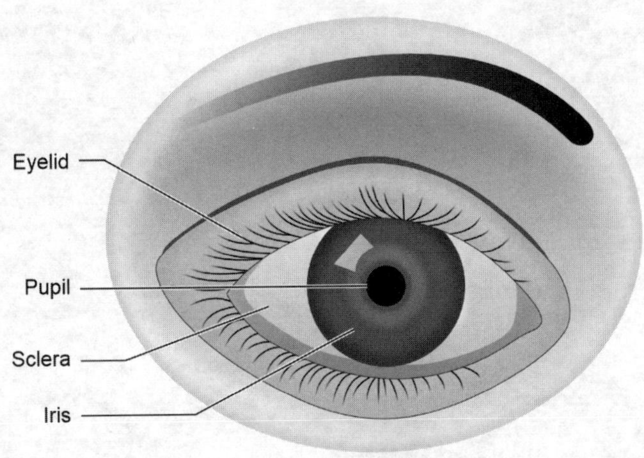

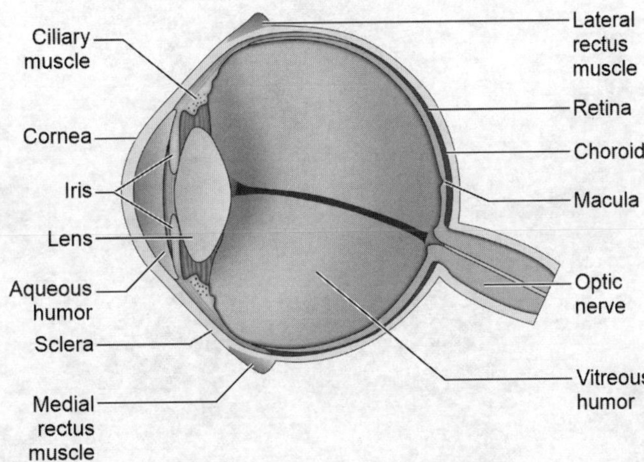

Eye Assessment

■ EVALUATION CRITERIA FOR EYE ASSESSMENT

Maximum Marks: 25

S. No.	Contents	Maximum marks	Allotted marks
1.	Patient's history	02	
2.	Ear internal examination	02	
3.	External eye examination	05	
4.	Ophthalmic examination	02	
5.	Complication and prognosis	05	
6.	Health teaching	05	
7.	Conclusion	04	
	Total	**25**	

Remarks:

Signature of Student   **Signature of Supervisor**

Patient's Identification Data

- Name :
- Age :
- Sex :
- Marital status :
- Hospital registration no. :
- Ward/bed no. :
- Address :
- Tel. no. :
- Religion :
- Education :
- Date of admission :
- Date of discharge :
- Diagnosis :
- Surgery :
- Date of surgery :
- Name of the doctor :
- Occupation :
- Monthly family income (₹) :
- Nursing alert :
- Sensitivity/allergy :
- Weight :
- Height :

Chief Complaints with Duration

Health History

Ask the patient the following:

- Vision loss
- Eye pain
- Double vision
- Eye tearing
- Dry eyes
- Eye drainage
- Eye appearance changes
- Blurred vision
- Have you noticed any changes in your vision
- Do you wear glasses or lenses
- Have you ever had surgery or injury
- Have you ever seen spots or floaters, flashes of light, or halos around the lights
- Do you a history of recurrent eye infection
- When was your last eye exam
- Do you have a history of HTN or diabetes
- What medications are currently taking
- Do you take any prescribed or OTC eye drops

Family History

S. No.	Name of family member	Age and sex	Relationship with patient	Occupation	Health status/ history of significant illness	Health habits

Family Tree

Socioeconomic History

- Occupation and social relationship:
- Monthly family income (₹):
- Health facility near home:
  - Type:
    - Hospital
    - Health center
    - Any other: If any other (specify)
  - Distance: __________ kms.
  - Transportation facility:
    - Yes
    - No
  - Housing: Type
    - Kutcha
    - Pucca
  - No. of rooms:
  - Toilet: Indian/western/temporary/open
  - Electricity: Yes/No
  - Drinking water source: Tap/well/pond/river/hand/pump

Dietary History

Health Habits: Functional Health Pattern

- Health perception/health management:
- Nutritional/metabolic:
- Elimination:
- Activity/exercise:
- Sleep/rest:
- Self-perception/self-concept:
- Role relationship:
- Sexuality/reproductive:
- Coping/stress–tolerance:
- Value/belief:
- Other comments/data:

Testing Visual Acuity

- Near sightedness:
- Far sightedness:
- Color vision:

Pupillary Response

Extraocular Movements

- Corneal light reflex test:

- Cardinal fields of gaze test:

External Eye Assessment

- General appearance:

- Eyelashes:

- Eyelids:

- Eyeball:

- Lacrimation gland and nasolacrimal gland:

- Conjunctiva:

- Sclera:

- Cornea and lenses:

- Iris:

- Pupils:

- Accommodation:

- Anterior chamber:

Performing Ophthalmic Examination

- Examine the retina:

- Blood vessels:

- Optic disc:

- Macula:

- Intraocular pressure:

Other Investigations

Date	Investigations done	Normal value	Patient value	Inference

Drug Study

S. No.	Drug trade name	Pharmacological name	Dose and frequency	Route	Action	Side effects and drug interaction	Nurses responsibility

Complications and Prognosis

Health Teaching

Summary and Conclusion

Case Study

EVALUATION CRITERIA FOR NURSING CASE STUDY

Maximum Marks: 100

S. No.	Contents	Maximum marks	Marks obtained
1.	Patient's history	04	
2.	Physical examination	04	
3.	Anatomy and physiology	05	
4.	Incidence and etiology	05	
5.	Pathophysiology	05	
6.	Clinical manifestations	06	
7.	Investigations	04	
8.	Complication and prognosis	05	
9.	Management: Medical and surgical	12	
10.	Drug study	10	
11.	Nursing care plan	15	
12.	Nurses' notes	08	
13.	Health education	06	
14.	Discharge planning	05	
15.	Conclusion and research evidence	03	
16.	Bibliography	03	
	Total	**100**	

Remarks:

Signature of Student   **Signature of Supervisor**

Introduction

Purposes of the Study

Objectives of the Study

Duration of the Study

Patient's Identification Data

- Name :
- Age :
- Sex :
- Marital status :
- Hospital registration no. :
- Ward/bed no. :
- Address :
- Tel. no. :
- Religion :
- Education :
- Date of admission :
- Date of discharge :
- Diagnosis :
- Operation :
- Date of operation :
- Name of the doctor :
- Occupation :
- Monthly family income (₹) :
- Nursing alert :
- Sensitivity/allergy/precaution :
- Weight :
- Height :

Informant

Information's relevant or not.

Chief Complaints with Duration

History of Present Illness

History of Past Medical Illness: Illness/medications/any restrictions.

History of Past Surgical Illness: Illness/medications/any restrictions.

Obstetrical History

Family History

S. No.	Name of family member	Age and sex	Relationship with patient	Occupation	Health status/ history of significant illness	Health habits

Family Tree

Socioeconomic History

- Occupation and social relationship:
- Monthly family income (₹):
- Health facility near home:
  - Type:
    - Hospital
    - Health center
    - Any other: If any other (specify)
  - Distance: __________ kms.
  - Transportation facility:
    - Yes
    - No
  - Housing: Type
    - Kutcha
    - Pucca
  - No. of rooms:
  - Toilet: Indian/western/temporary/open
  - Electricity: Yes/No
  - Drinking water source: Tap/well/pond/river/hand/pump

Dietary History

Health Habits: Functional Health Pattern

- Health perception/health management:

- Nutritional/metabolic:

- Elimination:

- Activity/exercise:

- Sleep/rest:

- Self-perception/self-concept:

- Role relationship:

- Sexuality/reproductive:

- Coping/stress–tolerance:

- Value/belief:

- Other comments/data:

Physical Examination

General Appearance

Height

Weight

Vital Signs

S. No.	Vital signs	Patient value	Normal value	Remarks
1.	Temperature			
2.	Pulse			
3.	Respiration			
4.	Blood pressure			

Head

- Scalp:
- Face:
- Sinus:
- Nodes:

Eyes

- Ocular movement:
- Pupils:
- Sclera:
- Cornea:

Ears

- External structures:
- Hearing:

Nose

- External structure:
- Septum:
- Mucous membrane:
- Patency:
- Olfactory sense:

Mouth

- Buccal mucosa:
- Gums:
- Teeth:
- Palates and uvula:
- Tonsillar area:
- Voice breath:

Neck

- Muscles:
- Trachea:
- Thyroid:
- Nodes:
- Vein distension:

Thorax

- Chest shape:
- Respiratory rate:
- Type of respiration:
- Thoracic expansion:
- Palpation:
- Percussion:
- Breath sounds:

Cardiovascular System

- Precordium—Inspection:
- Palpation:
- Auscultation:
- Apical rate and rhythm:

Central and Peripheral Vessels

- Carotid arteries:
- Peripheral pulses—Brachial:
- Radial:
- Femoral:
- Popliteal:
- Dorsal pedal:
- Posterior tibial:
- Capillary refill:

Abdomen

- Inspection:

- Auscultation:

- Percussion:

- Palpation:

Musculoskeletal System

- Gait:

- Upper extremities:

- Lower extremities:

- Muscle strength:

- Joints:

- Range of motion:

- Spine:

Nervous System

- Mental status:

  - Language:

  - Orientation:

  - Memory attention span:

- Level of consciousness (GCS):

- Cranial nerves:

- Deep tendon reflex:

- Gross and fine motor function of UE and LE:

- Sensory function:

  - Light touch:

  - Pain:

  - Temperature:

- Position:

Genitalia and Rectal Examination

- Inspection:

- Palpation:

Comparison of the Patient's Disease with Book Picture

- Definition

- Anatomy and physiology

- Incidence

- Etiology

Book picture	Patient picture

- Pathophysiology

- Signs and symptoms

- Diagnosis provisional and final

Book picture	Patient picture

Investigations

Date	Investigations done	Normal value	Patient value	Inference

Management: Medical or Surgical

Drug Study

S. No.	Drug trade name	Pharmacological name	Dose and frequency	Route	Action	Side effects and drug interaction	Nurses responsibility

Nursing Care Plan

Nursing assessment: Subjective and objective data	Nursing diagnosis	Goals	Nursing intervention		Rationale	Evaluation
			Planned	Implemented		

Nurses' Notes

Time	Medication	Diet/nutrition	Observation/intervention/evaluation	Signature

Complications and Prognosis

Health Teaching

Summary and Conclusion

Bibliography

Case Presentation

EVALUATION CRITERIA FOR NURSING CASE PRESENTATION

Maximum Marks: 100

S. No.	Contents	Maximum marks	Marks obtained
1.	Assessment	10	
2.	Co-relation with patient and book	15	
3.	Drug study	06	
4.	Nursing care plan	25	
5.	Nurses' notes	05	
6.	Health education	06	
7.	Use of AV aids	08	
8.	Physical arrangement	05	
9.	Group participation	10	
10.	Effectiveness of presentation	05	
11.	Bibliography	05	
	Total	**100**	

Remarks:

Signature of Student   **Signature of Supervisor**

Patient's Identification Data

- Name :
- Age :
- Sex :
- Marital status :
- Hospital registration no. :
- Ward/bed no. :
- Address :
- Tel. no. :
- Religion :
- Education :
- Date of admission :
- Date of discharge :
- Diagnosis :
- Operation :
- Date of operation :
- Name of the doctor :
- Occupation :
- Monthly family income (₹) :
- Nursing alert :
- Sensitivity/allergy/precaution :
- Weight :
- Height :

Informant

Information's relevant or not.

Chief Complaints with Duration

History of Present Illness

History of Past Medical Illness: Illness/medications/any restrictions.

History of Past Surgical Illness: Illness/medications/any restrictions.

Obstetrical History

Family History

S. No.	Name of family member	Age and sex	Relationship with patient	Occupation	Health status/ history of significant illness	Health habits

Family Tree

Socioeconomic History

- Occupation and social relationship:
- Monthly family income (₹):
- Health facility near home:
  - Type:
    - Hospital
    - Health center
    - Any other: If any other (specify)
  - Distance: __________ kms.
  - Transportation facility:
    - Yes
    - No
  - Housing: Type
    - Kutcha
    - Pucca
  - No. of rooms:
  - Toilet: Indian/western/temporary/open
  - Electricity: Yes/No
  - Drinking water source: Tap/well/pond/river/hand/pump

Dietary History

Health Habits: Functional Health Pattern

- Health perception/health management:

- Nutritional/metabolic:

- Elimination:

- Activity/exercise:

- Sleep/rest:

- Self-perception/self-concept:

- Role relationship:

- Sexuality/reproductive:

- Coping/stress–tolerance:

- Value/belief:

- Other comments/data:

Physical Examination

General Appearance

Height

Weight

Vital Signs

S. No.	Vital signs	Patient value	Normal value	Remarks
1.	Temperature			
2.	Pulse			
3.	Respiration			
4.	Blood pressure			

Head

- Scalp:
- Face:
- Sinus:
- Nodes:

Eyes

- Ocular movement:
- Pupils:
- Sclera:
- Cornea:

Ears

- External structures:
- Hearing:

Nose

- External structure:
- Septum:
- Mucous membrane:
- Patency:
- Olfactory sense:

Mouth

- Buccal mucosa:
- Gums:
- Teeth:
- Palates and uvula:
- Tonsillar area:
- Voice breath:

Neck

- Muscles:
- Trachea:
- Thyroid:
- Nodes:
- Vein distension:

Thorax

- Chest shape:
- Respiratory rate:
- Type of respiration:
- Thoracic expansion:
- Palpation:
- Percussion:
- Breath sounds:

Cardiovascular System

- Precordium—Inspection:
- Palpation:
- Auscultation:
- Apical rate and rhythm:

Central and Peripheral Vessels

- Carotid arteries:
- Peripheral pulses—Brachial:
- Radial:
- Femoral:
- Popliteal:
- Dorsal pedal:
- Posterior tibial:
- Capillary refill:

Abdomen

- Inspection:
- Auscultation:
- Percussion:
- Palpation:

Musculoskeletal System

- Gait:
- Upper extremities:
- Lower extremities:
- Muscle strength:
- Joints:
- Range of motion:
- Spine:

Nervous System

- Mental status:
  - Language:
  - Orientation:
  - Memory attention span:
- Level of consciousness (GCS):
- Cranial nerves:
- Deep tendon reflex:
- Gross and fine motor function of UE and LE:
- Sensory function:
  - Light touch:
  - Pain:
  - Temperature:
- Position:

Genitalia and Rectal Examination

- Inspection:
- Palpation:

Comparison of the Patient's Disease with Book Picture

- Anatomy and physiology

- Incidence

- Etiology

S. No.	Book picture	Patient picture

- Pathophysiology

- Clinical manifestations

S. No.	Book picture	Patient picture

- Diagnosis provisional and final

S. No.	Book picture	Patient picture

Investigations

Date	Investigations done	Normal value	Patient value	Inference

Management: Medical or Surgical

Drug Study

S. No.	Drug trade name	Pharmacological name	Dose and frequency	Route	Action	Side effects and drug interaction	Nurses responsibility

Nursing Care Plan

Nursing assessment: Subjective and objective data	Nursing diagnosis	Goals	Nursing intervention		Rationale	Evaluation
			Planned	Implemented		

Nurses' Notes

Time	Medication	Diet/nutrition	Observation/ intervention/evaluation	Signature

Complications and Prognosis

Health Teaching

Discharge Planning/Notes

Summary and Conclusion

Bibliography

Health Teaching

■ **EVALUATION CRITERIA FOR HEALTH TEACHING**

- Name of the institution :
- Name of the student :
- Language :
- Topic :
- Audience :
- Ward/field :
- Name of the supervisor/teacher :   Date:

S. No.	Criteria	Marks allotted	Marks obtained
	Content		
1.	Lesson planning	05	
2.	Appropriateness, relevancy and adequacy of content	08	
3.	Organization	04	
4.	Up to date and evidence based	03	
	Presentation		
1.	Physical arrangement	03	
2.	Communication skill	05	
3.	Confidence	03	
4.	Group involvement	03	
	AV Aids		
1.	Selection and preparation	04	
2.	Effective use of AV Aids	03	
	Other		
1.	Time management	03	
2.	Acceptance of guidance	03	
3.	Reference	03	
	Total	**50**	

Signature of Student   **Signature of Supervisor**

Health Education

Topic Selected

- Name of the student teacher   :

- Name of the supervisor   :

- Venue   :

- Date   :

- Time   :

- Group   :

- Previous knowledge of the group   :

- AV aids used   :

- General objectives:

- Specific objectives:

Lesson Plan for Health Talk

S. No.	Time	Specific objectives	Contents	Teaching-learning activities	AV Aids	Evaluation

Nursing Management of Patients with Kidney and Urinary System Disorders

- ☑ Renal and Urinary System Assessment
- ☑ Case Study
- ☑ Case Presentation
- ☑ Drug Presentation

Anatomical Diagram of Urinary System

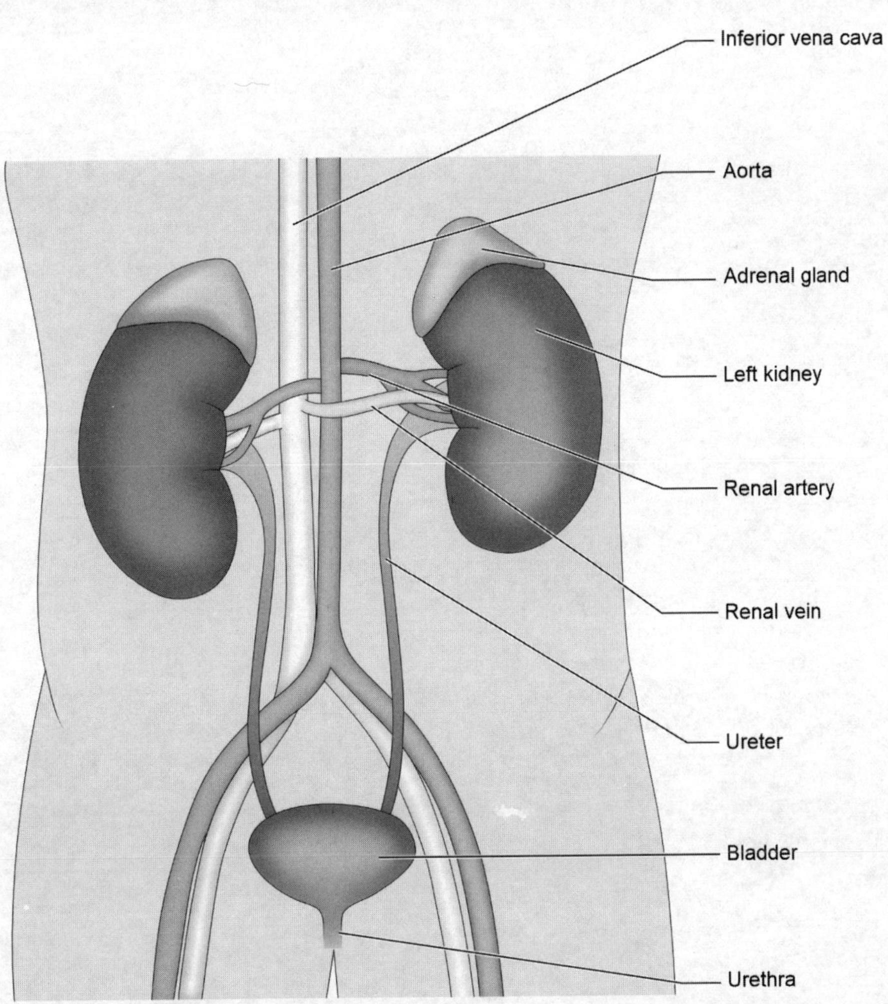

Renal and Urinary System Assessment

EVALUATION CRITERIA FOR RENAL AND URINARY ASSESSMENT

Maximum Marks: 25

S. No.	Contents	Maximum marks	Allotted marks
1.	Patient's history	02	
2.	Abdominal assessment	03	
3.	Kidney and urinary assessment	05	
4.	Complication and prognosis	03	
5.	Health teaching	03	
6.	Conclusion	03	
	Total	**25**	

Remarks:

Signature of Student   **Signature of Supervisor**

Patient's Identification Data

- Name :
- Age :
- Sex :
- Marital status :
- Hospital registration no. :
- Ward/bed no. :
- Address :
- Tel. no. :
- Religion :
- Education :
- Date of admission :
- Date of discharge :
- Diagnosis :
- Operation :
- Date of operation :
- Name of the doctor :
- Occupation :
- Monthly family income (₹) :
- Nursing alert :
- Sensitivity/allergy/precaution :
- Weight :
- Height :

Informant

Information's relevant or not.

Chief Complaints with Duration

History of Present Illness

History of Urinary Tract Infection/Kidney Stone

History of Past Surgical Illness: Illness/medications/any restrictions.

Family History

S. No.	Name of family member	Age and sex	Relationship with patient	Occupation	Health status/ history of significant illness	Health habits

Family Tree

Socioeconomic History

- Occupation and social relationship:
- Monthly family income (₹):
- Health facility near home:
  - Type:
    - ◆ Hospital
    - ◆ Health center
    - ◆ Any other: If any other (specify)
  - Distance: ___________ kms.
  - Transportation facility:
    - ◆ Yes
    - ◆ No
  - Housing: Type
    - ◆ Kutcha
    - ◆ Pucca
  - No. of rooms:
  - Toilet: Indian/western/temporary/open
  - Electricity: Yes/No
  - Drinking water source: Tap/well/pond/river/hand/pump

Dietary History

Health Habits: Functional Health Pattern

- Health perception/health management:

- Nutritional/metabolic:

- Elimination:

- Activity/exercise:

- Sleep/rest:

- Self-perception/self-concept:

- Role relationship:

- Sexuality/reproductive:

- Coping/stress–tolerance:

- Value/belief:

- Other comments/data:

Kidney and Urinary Tract Assessment

General Appearance

Vital Signs

S. No.	Vital signs	Patient value	Normal value	Remarks
1.	Temperature			
2.	Pulse			
3.	Respiration			
4.	Blood pressure			

Abdominal Assessment

- Inspection:
- Auscultation:
- Palpation:

Kidney Assessment

- Percussion:
- Palpation:

Bladder Assessment: Palpation

- Flanks area:

- Genitalia (discharge or lesion):

- Assessment of peripheral edema (legs/ankles):

Diagnostic Assessment

Blood Test

- Serum creatinine:

- Blood urea nitrogen:

- Urinalysis:

- Specific gravity:

- Ketone bodies:

Urine Test

- Urinalysis:

- Protein:

- Culture and sensitivity:

- Creatinine clearance test:

- Urine electrolytes:

- Osmolality:

Radiographic Test

- KUB X-Ray:

- Intravenous urography:

- Cystography and cystoscopy:

- USG:

- Renal scan:

- Renal arteriography:

- Voiding cystourethrography:

Additional Assessment

- Pain assessment:

- Fluid intake and output:

Drug Study

S. No.	Drug trade name	Pharmacological name	Dose and frequency	Route	Action	Side effects and drug interaction	Nurses responsibility

Complications and Prognosis

Health Teaching

Summary and Conclusion

Case Study

▌EVALUATION CRITERIA FOR NURSING CASE STUDY

Maximum Marks: 100

S. No.	Contents	Maximum marks	Marks obtained
1.	Patient's history	04	
2.	Physical examination	04	
3.	Anatomy and physiology	05	
4.	Incidence and etiology	05	
5.	Pathophysiology	05	
6.	Clinical manifestations	06	
7.	Investigations	04	
8.	Complication and prognosis	05	
9.	Management: Medical and surgical	12	
10.	Drug study	10	
11.	Nursing care plan	15	
12.	Nurses' notes	08	
13.	Health education	06	
14.	Discharge planning	05	
15.	Conclusion and research evidence	03	
16.	Bibliography	03	
	Total	**100**	

Remarks:

Signature of Student

Signature of Supervisor

Introduction

Purposes of the Study

Objectives of the Study

Duration of the Study

Patient's Identification Data

- Name :
- Age :
- Sex :
- Marital status :
- Hospital registration no. :
- Ward/bed no. :
- Address :
- Tel. no. :
- Religion :
- Education :
- Date of admission :
- Date of discharge :
- Diagnosis :
- Operation :
- Date of operation :
- Name of the doctor :
- Occupation :
- Monthly family income (₹) :
- Nursing alert :
- Sensitivity/allergy/precaution :
- Weight :
- Height :

Informant

Information's relevant or not.

Chief Complaints with Duration

History of Present Illness

History of Past Medical Illness: Illness/medications/any restrictions.

History of Past Surgical Illness: Illness/medications/any restrictions.

Obstetrical History

Family History

S. No.	Name of family member	Age and sex	Relationship with patient	Occupation	Health status/ history of significant illness	Health habits

Family Tree

Socioeconomic History

- Occupation and social relationship:
- Monthly family income (₹):
- Health facility near home:
  - Type:
    - Hospital
    - Health center
    - Any other: If any other (specify)
  - Distance: __________ kms.
  - Transportation facility:
    - Yes
    - No
  - Housing: Type
    - Kutcha
    - Pucca
  - No. of rooms:
  - Toilet: Indian/western/temporary/open
  - Electricity: Yes/No
  - Drinking water source: Tap/well/pond/river/hand/pump

Dietary History

Health Habits: Functional Health Pattern

- Health perception/health management:

- Nutritional/metabolic:

- Elimination:

- Activity/exercise:

- Sleep/rest:

- Self-perception/self-concept:

- Role relationship:

- Sexuality/reproductive:

- Coping/stress–tolerance:

- Value/belief:

- Other comments/data:

Physical Examination

General Appearance

Height

Weight

Vital Signs

S. No.	Vital signs	Patient value	Normal value	Remarks
1.	Temperature			
2.	Pulse			
3.	Respiration			
4.	Blood pressure			

Head

- Scalp:
- Face:
- Sinus:
- Nodes:

Eyes

- Ocular movement:
- Pupils:
- Sclera:
- Cornea:

Ears

- External structures:
- Hearing:

Nose

- External structure:
- Septum:
- Mucous membrane:
- Patency:
- Olfactory sense:

Mouth

- Buccal mucosa:
- Gums:
- Teeth:
- Palates and uvula:
- Tonsillar area:
- Voice breath:

Neck

- Muscles:
- Trachea:
- Thyroid:
- Nodes:
- Vein distension:

Thorax

- Chest shape:
- Respiratory rate:
- Type of respiration:
- Thoracic expansion:
- Palpation:
- Percussion:
- Breath sounds:

Cardiovascular System

- Precordium—Inspection:
- Palpation:
- Auscultation:
- Apical rate and rhythm:

Central and Peripheral Vessels

- Carotid arteries:
- Peripheral pulses—Brachial:
- Radial:
- Femoral:
- Popliteal:
- Dorsal pedal:
- Posterior tibial:
- Capillary refill:

Abdomen

- Inspection:
- Auscultation:
- Percussion:
- Palpation:

Musculoskeletal System

- Gait:
- Upper extremities:
- Lower extremities:
- Muscle strength:
- Joints:
- Range of motion:
- Spine:

Nervous System

- Mental status:
  - Language:
  - Orientation:
  - Memory attention span:
- Level of consciousness (GCS):
- Cranial nerves:
- Deep tendon reflex:
- Gross and fine motor function of UE and LE:
- Sensory function:
  - Light touch:
  - Pain:
  - Temperature:
- Position:

Genitalia and Rectal Examination

- Inspection:
- Palpation:

Comparison of the Patient's Disease with Book Picture

- Definition

- Anatomy and physiology

- Incidence

- Etiology

Book picture	Patient picture

- Pathophysiology

- Signs and symptoms

- Diagnosis provisional and final

Book picture	Patient picture

Investigations

Date	Investigations done	Normal value	Patient value	Inference

Management: Medical or Surgical

Drug Study

S. No.	Drug trade name	Pharmacological name	Dose and frequency	Route	Action	Side effects and drug interaction	Nurses responsibility

Nursing Care Plan

Nursing assessment: Subjective and objective data	Nursing diagnosis	Goals	Nursing intervention		Rationale	Evaluation
			Planned	Implemented		

Nurses' Notes

Time	Medication	Diet/nutrition	Observation/ intervention/evaluation	Signature

Complications and Prognosis

Health Teaching

Summary and Conclusion

Bibliography

Case Presentation

▮ EVALUATION CRITERIA FOR NURSING CASE PRESENTATION

Maximum Marks: 100

S. No.	Contents	Maximum marks	Marks obtained
1.	Assessment	10	
2.	Co-relation with patient and book	15	
3.	Drug study	06	
4.	Nursing care plan	25	
5.	Nurses' notes	05	
6.	Health education	06	
7.	Use of AV aids	08	
8.	Physical arrangement	05	
9.	Group participation	10	
10.	Effectiveness of presentation	05	
11.	Bibliography	05	
	Total	**100**	

Remarks:

Signature of Student   **Signature of Supervisor**

Patient's Identification Data

- Name :
- Age :
- Sex :
- Marital status :
- Hospital registration no. :
- Ward/bed no. :
- Address :
- Tel. no. :
- Religion :
- Education :
- Date of admission :
- Date of discharge :
- Diagnosis :
- Operation :
- Date of operation :
- Name of the doctor :
- Occupation :
- Monthly family income (₹) :
- Nursing alert :
- Sensitivity/allergy/precaution :
- Weight :
- Height :

Informant

Information's relevant or not.

Chief Complaints with Duration

History of Present Illness

History of Past Medical Illness: Illness/medications/any restrictions.

History of Past Surgical Illness: Illness/medications/any restrictions.

Obstetrical History

Family History

S. No.	Name of family member	Age and sex	Relationship with patient	Occupation	Health status/ history of significant illness	Health habits

Family Tree

Socioeconomic History

- Occupation and social relationship:
- Monthly family income (₹):
- Health facility near home:
  - Type:
    - Hospital
    - Health center
    - Any other: If any other (specify)
  - Distance: __________ kms.
  - Transportation facility:
    - Yes
    - No
  - Housing: Type
    - Kutcha
    - Pucca
  - No. of rooms:
  - Toilet: Indian/western/temporary/open
  - Electricity: Yes/No
  - Drinking water source: Tap/well/pond/river/hand/pump

Dietary History

Health Habits: Functional Health Pattern

- Health perception/health management:

- Nutritional/metabolic:

- Elimination:

- Activity/exercise:

- Sleep/rest:

- Self-perception/self-concept:

- Role relationship:

- Sexuality/reproductive:

- Coping/stress–tolerance:

- Value/belief:

- Other comments/data:

Physical Examination

General Appearance

Height

Weight

Vital Signs

S. No.	Vital signs	Patient value	Normal value	Remarks
1.	Temperature			
2.	Pulse			
3.	Respiration			
4.	Blood pressure			

Head

- Scalp:
- Face:
- Sinus:
- Nodes:

Eyes

- Ocular movement:
- Pupils:
- Sclera:
- Cornea:

Ears

- External structures:
- Hearing:

Nose

- External structure:
- Septum:
- Mucous membrane:
- Patency:
- Olfactory sense:

Mouth

- Buccal mucosa:
- Gums:
- Teeth:
- Palates and uvula:
- Tonsillar area:
- Voice breath:

Neck

- Muscles:
- Trachea:
- Thyroid:
- Nodes:
- Vein distension:

Thorax

- Chest shape:
- Respiratory rate:
- Type of respiration:
- Thoracic expansion:
- Palpation:
- Percussion:
- Breath sounds:

Cardiovascular System

- Precordium—Inspection:
- Palpation:
- Auscultation:
- Apical rate and rhythm:

Central and Peripheral Vessels

- Carotid arteries:
- Peripheral pulses—Brachial:
- Radial:
- Femoral:
- Popliteal:
- Dorsal pedal:
- Posterior tibial:
- Capillary refill:

Abdomen

- Inspection:
- Auscultation:
- Percussion:
- Palpation:

Musculoskeletal System

- Gait:
- Upper extremities:
- Lower extremities:
- Muscle strength:
- Joints:
- Range of motion:
- Spine:

Nervous System

- Mental status:
  - Language:
  - Orientation:
  - Memory attention span:
- Level of consciousness (GCS):
- Cranial nerves:
- Deep tendon reflex:
- Gross and fine motor function of UE and LE:
- Sensory function:
  - Light touch:
  - Pain:
  - Temperature:
- Position:

Genitalia and Rectal Examination

- Inspection:
- Palpation:

Comparison of the Patient's Disease with Book Picture

- Anatomy and physiology

- Incidence

- Etiology

S. No.	Book picture	Patient picture

- Pathophysiology

- Clinical manifestations

S. No.	Book picture	Patient picture

- Diagnosis provisional and final

S. No.	Book picture	Patient picture

Investigations

Date	Investigations done	Normal value	Patient value	Inference

Management: Medical or Surgical

Drug Study

S. No.	Drug trade name	Pharmacological name	Dose and frequency	Route	Action	Side effects and drug interaction	Nurses responsibility

Nursing Care Plan

Nursing assessment: Subjective and objective data	Nursing diagnosis	Goals	Nursing intervention		Rationale	Evaluation
			Planned	Implemented		

Nurses' Notes

Time	Medication	Diet/nutrition	Observation/ intervention/evaluation	Signature

Complications and Prognosis

Health Teaching

Discharge Planning/Notes

Summary and Conclusion

Bibliography

Drug Presentation

EVALUATION CRITERIA FOR DRUG PRESENTATION

Maximum Marks: 25

S. No.	Contents	Maximum marks	Marks obtained
1.	Name of drug	02	
2.	Dose, time and route	02	
3.	Action	03	
4.	Indication	03	
5.	Contraindication	03	
6.	Side-effects	03	
7.	Nursing responsibilities	07	
8.	Conclusion	02	
	Total	**25**	

Remarks:

Signature of Student   **Signature of Supervisor**

Introduction

Drug Name and Classification

Indication

Mechanism of Action

Dosage and Administration

Side Effects and Adverse Reactions

Contraindication and Precautions

Drug Interactions

Patient Education

Nursing Responsibility

Conclusion

Bibliography

Nursing Management of Patients with Burns and Reconstructive Surgery

- ☑ Burn Wound Assessment
- ☑ Case Study
- ☑ Case Presentation

Burn Wound Assessment

EVALUATION CRITERIA FOR BURN ASSESSMENT

Maximum Marks: 25

S. No.	Contents	Maximum marks	Marks obtained
1.	Patient's history	02	
2.	Initial burn assessment	05	
3.	Assessment of burn severity and depth	05	
4.	Fluid resuscitation	05	
5.	Complication and prognosis	03	
6.	Health teaching	02	
7.	Conclusion	03	
	Total	**25**	

Remarks:

Signature of Student   **Signature of Supervisor**

Patient's Identification Data

- Name   :
- Age   :
- Sex   :
- Marital status   :
- Hospital registration no.   :
- Ward/bed no.   :
- Address   :
- Tel. no.   :
- Religion   :
- Education   :
- Date of admission   :
- Date of discharge   :
- Diagnosis   :
- Operation   :
- Date of operation   :
- Name of the doctor   :
- Occupation   :
- Monthly family income (₹)   :
- Nursing alert   :
- Sensitivity/allergy/precaution :
- Weight   :
- Height   :

Informant

Information's relevant or not.

Burn Assessment

Type of burn:

Initial Assessment

Airway:

Breathing:

Circulation:

Disability:

Exposure:

Assessing Burn Depth

First degree burn:

Second degree burn:

Third degree burn:

Fourth degree burn:

Assessing the Burn Severity

Wallace's rule of nine:

Rule of palm:

Lund and browder chart:

Location of Burn

Associated Injuries or Conditions

Sign of infection

Patient Medical History (if Any)

Fluid Resuscitation

Parkland formula:

Evans formula:

Brooke formula:

Modified Brooke formula:

Monitoring of Resuscitation

Urine output:

Blood pressure:

Heart rate:

Hematocrit and hemoglobin:

Drug Study

S. No.	Drug trade name	Pharmacological name	Dose and frequency	Route	Action	Side effects and drug interaction	Nurses responsibility

Complications and Prognosis

Health Teaching

Summary and Conclusion

Case Study

EVALUATION CRITERIA FOR NURSING CASE STUDY

Maximum Marks: 100

S. No.	Contents	Maximum marks	Marks obtained
1.	Patient's history	04	
2.	Physical examination	04	
3.	Anatomy and physiology	05	
4.	Incidence and etiology	05	
5.	Pathophysiology	05	
6.	Clinical manifestations	06	
7.	Investigations	04	
8.	Complication and prognosis	05	
9.	Management: Medical and surgical	12	
10.	Drug study	10	
11.	Nursing care plan	15	
12.	Nurses' notes	08	
13.	Health education	06	
14.	Discharge planning	05	
15.	Conclusion and research evidence	03	
16.	Bibliography	03	
	Total	**100**	

Remarks:

Signature of Student **Signature of Supervisor**

Introduction

Purposes of the Study

Objectives of the Study

Duration of the Study

Patient's Identification Data

- Name :
- Age :
- Sex :
- Marital status :
- Hospital registration no. :
- Ward/bed no. :
- Address :
- Tel. no. :
- Religion :
- Education :
- Date of admission :
- Date of discharge :
- Diagnosis :
- Operation :
- Date of operation :
- Name of the doctor :
- Occupation :
- Monthly family income (₹) :
- Nursing alert :
- Sensitivity/allergy/precaution :
- Weight :
- Height :

Informant

Information's relevant or not.

Chief Complaints with Duration

History of Present Illness

History of Past Medical Illness: Illness/medications/any restrictions.

History of Past Surgical Illness: Illness/medications/any restrictions.

Obstetrical History

Family History

S. No.	Name of family member	Age and sex	Relationship with patient	Occupation	Health status/ history of significant illness	Health habits

Family Tree

Socioeconomic History

- Occupation and social relationship:
- Monthly family income (₹):
- Health facility near home:
  - Type:
    - Hospital
    - Health center
    - Any other: If any other (specify)
  - Distance: _________ kms.
  - Transportation facility:
    - Yes
    - No
  - Housing: Type
    - Kutcha
    - Pucca
  - No. of rooms:
  - Toilet: Indian/western/temporary/open
  - Electricity: Yes/No
  - Drinking water source: Tap/well/pond/river/hand/pump

Dietary History

Health Habits: Functional Health Pattern

- Health perception/health management:

- Nutritional/metabolic:

- Elimination:

- Activity/exercise:

- Sleep/rest:

- Self-perception/self-concept:

- Role relationship:

- Sexuality/reproductive:

- Coping/stress–tolerance:

- Value/belief:

- Other comments/data:

Physical Examination

General Appearance

Height

Weight

Vital Signs

S. No.	Vital signs	Patient value	Normal value	Remarks
1.	Temperature			
2.	Pulse			
3.	Respiration			
4.	Blood pressure			

Head

- Scalp:
- Face:
- Sinus:
- Nodes:

Eyes

- Ocular movement:
- Pupils:
- Sclera:
- Cornea:

Ears

- External structures:
- Hearing:

Nose

- External structure:
- Septum:
- Mucous membrane:
- Patency:
- Olfactory sense:

Mouth

- Buccal mucosa:
- Gums:
- Teeth:
- Palates and uvula:
- Tonsillar area:
- Voice breath:

Neck

- Muscles:
- Trachea:
- Thyroid:
- Nodes:
- Vein distension:

Thorax

- Chest shape:
- Respiratory rate:
- Type of respiration:
- Thoracic expansion:
- Palpation:
- Percussion:
- Breath sounds:

Cardiovascular System

- Precordium—Inspection:
- Palpation:
- Auscultation:
- Apical rate and rhythm:

Central and Peripheral Vessels

- Carotid arteries:
- Peripheral pulses—Brachial:
- Radial:
- Femoral:
- Popliteal:
- Dorsal pedal:
- Posterior tibial:
- Capillary refill:

Abdomen

- Inspection:

- Auscultation:

- Percussion:

- Palpation:

Musculoskeletal System

- Gait:

- Upper extremities:

- Lower extremities:

- Muscle strength:

- Joints:

- Range of motion:

- Spine:

Nervous System

- Mental status:

  - Language:

  - Orientation:

  - Memory attention span:

- Level of consciousness (GCS):

- Cranial nerves:

- Deep tendon reflex:

- Gross and fine motor function of UE and LE:

- Sensory function:

  - Light touch:

  - Pain:

  - Temperature:

- Position:

Genitalia and Rectal Examination

- Inspection:

- Palpation:

Comparison of the Patient's Disease with Book Picture

- Definition

- Anatomy and physiology

- Incidence

- Etiology

Book picture	Patient picture

- Pathophysiology

- Signs and symptoms

- Diagnosis provisional and final

Book picture	Patient picture

Investigations

Date	Investigations done	Normal value	Patient value	Inference

Management: Medical or Surgical

Drug Study

S. No.	Drug trade name	Pharmacological name	Dose and frequency	Route	Action	Side effects and drug interaction	Nurses responsibility

Nursing Care Plan

Nursing assessment: Subjective and objective data	Nursing diagnosis	Goals	Nursing intervention		Rationale	Evaluation
			Planned	Implemented		

Nurses' Notes

Time	Medication	Diet/nutrition	Observation/intervention/evaluation	Signature

Complications and Prognosis

Health Teaching

Summary and Conclusion

Bibliography

Case Presentation

■ EVALUATION CRITERIA FOR NURSING CASE PRESENTATION

Maximum Marks: 100

S. No.	Contents	Maximum marks	Marks obtained
1.	Assessment	10	
2.	Co-relation with patient and book	15	
3.	Drug study	06	
4.	Nursing care plan	25	
5.	Nurses' notes	05	
6.	Health education	06	
7.	Use of AV aids	08	
8.	Physical arrangement	05	
9.	Group participation	10	
10.	Effectiveness of presentation	05	
11.	Bibliography	05	
	Total	**100**	

Remarks:

Signature of Student   **Signature of Supervisor**

Patient's Identification Data

- Name :
- Age :
- Sex :
- Marital status :
- Hospital registration no. :
- Ward/bed no. :
- Address :
- Tel. no. :
- Religion :
- Education :
- Date of admission :
- Date of discharge :
- Diagnosis :
- Operation :
- Date of operation :
- Name of the doctor :
- Occupation :
- Monthly family income (₹) :
- Nursing alert :
- Sensitivity/allergy/precaution :
- Weight :
- Height :

Informant

Information's relevant or not.

Chief Complaints with Duration

History of Present Illness

History of Past Medical Illness: Illness/medications/any restrictions.

History of Past Surgical Illness: Illness/medications/any restrictions.

Obstetrical History

Family History

S. No.	Name of family member	Age and sex	Relationship with patient	Occupation	Health status/ history of significant illness	Health habits

Family Tree

Socioeconomic History

- Occupation and social relationship:
- Monthly family income (₹):
- Health facility near home:
  - Type:
    - Hospital
    - Health center
    - Any other: If any other (specify)
  - Distance: __________ kms.
  - Transportation facility:
    - Yes
    - No
  - Housing: Type
    - Kutcha
    - Pucca
  - No. of rooms:
  - Toilet: Indian/western/temporary/open
  - Electricity: Yes/No
  - Drinking water source: Tap/well/pond/river/hand/pump

Dietary History

Health Habits: Functional Health Pattern

- Health perception/health management:

- Nutritional/metabolic:

- Elimination:

- Activity/exercise:

- Sleep/rest:

- Self-perception/self-concept:

- Role relationship:

- Sexuality/reproductive:

- Coping/stress–tolerance:

- Value/belief:

- Other comments/data:

Physical Examination

General Appearance

Height

Weight

Vital Signs

S. No.	Vital signs	Patient value	Normal value	Remarks
1.	Temperature			
2.	Pulse			
3.	Respiration			
4.	Blood pressure			

Head

- Scalp:
- Face:
- Sinus:
- Nodes:

Eyes

- Ocular movement:
- Pupils:
- Sclera:
- Cornea:

Ears

- External structures:
- Hearing:

Nose

- External structure:
- Septum:
- Mucous membrane:
- Patency:
- Olfactory sense:

Mouth

- Buccal mucosa:
- Gums:
- Teeth:
- Palates and uvula:
- Tonsillar area:
- Voice breath:

Neck

- Muscles:
- Trachea:
- Thyroid:
- Nodes:
- Vein distension:

Thorax

- Chest shape:
- Respiratory rate:
- Type of respiration:
- Thoracic expansion:
- Palpation:
- Percussion:
- Breath sounds:

Cardiovascular System

- Precordium—Inspection:
- Palpation:
- Auscultation:
- Apical rate and rhythm:

Central and Peripheral Vessels

- Carotid arteries:
- Peripheral pulses—Brachial:
- Radial:
- Femoral:
- Popliteal:
- Dorsal pedal:
- Posterior tibial:
- Capillary refill:

Abdomen

- Inspection:

- Auscultation:

- Percussion:

- Palpation:

Musculoskeletal System

- Gait:

- Upper extremities:

- Lower extremities:

- Muscle strength:

- Joints:

- Range of motion:

- Spine:

Nervous System

- Mental status:

  - Language:

  - Orientation:

  - Memory attention span:

- Level of consciousness (GCS):

- Cranial nerves:

- Deep tendon reflex:

- Gross and fine motor function of UE and LE:

- Sensory function:

  - Light touch:

  - Pain:

  - Temperature:

- Position:

Genitalia and Rectal Examination

- Inspection:

- Palpation:

Comparison of the Patient's Disease with Book Picture

- Anatomy and physiology

- Incidence

- Etiology

S. No.	Book picture	Patient picture

- Pathophysiology

- Clinical manifestations

S. No.	Book picture	Patient picture

- Diagnosis provisional and final

S. No.	Book picture	Patient picture

Investigations

Date	Investigations done	Normal value	Patient value	Inference

Management: Medical or Surgical

Drug Study

S. No.	Drug trade name	Pharmacological name	Dose and frequency	Route	Action	Side effects and drug interaction	Nurses responsibility

Nursing Care Plan

Nursing assessment: Subjective and objective data	Nursing diagnosis	Goals	Nursing intervention		Rationale	Evaluation
			Planned	Implemented		

Nurses' Notes

Time	Medication	Diet/nutrition	Observation/ intervention/evaluation	Signature

Complications and Prognosis

Health Teaching

Discharge Planning/Notes

Summary and Conclusion

Bibliography

Nursing Management of Patients with Neurological Disorders

- ☑ Neurological Assessment
- ☑ Case Study
- ☑ Case Presentation
- ☑ Drug Presentation

Anatomical Diagram of Nervous System

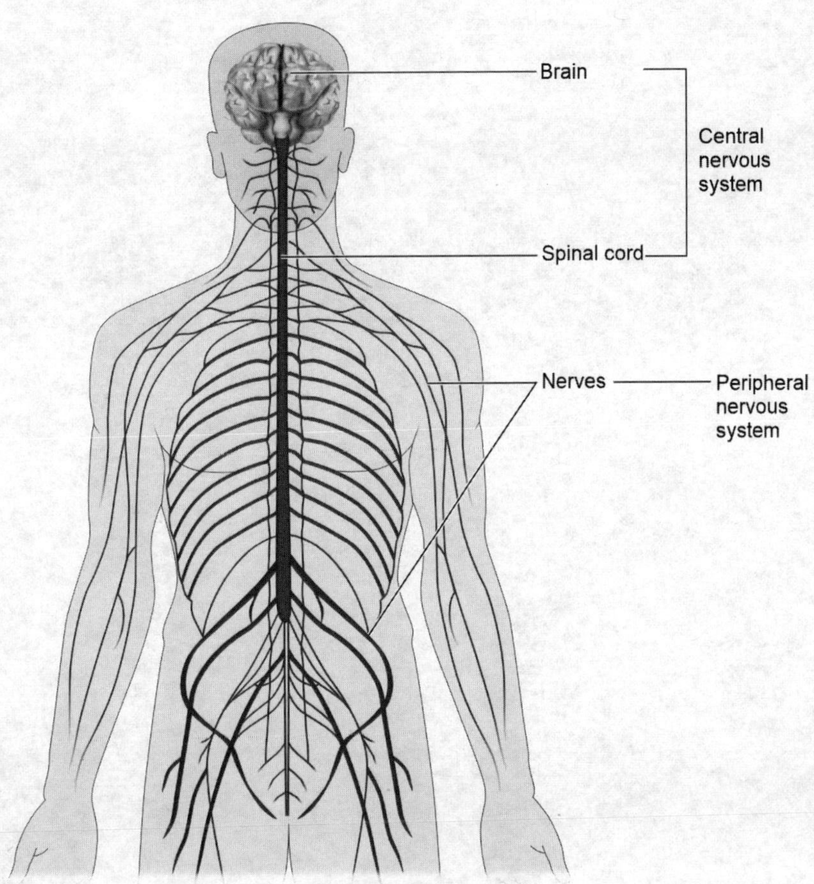

Neurological Assessment

▌EVALUATION CRITERIA FOR NEUROLOGICAL ASSESSMENT

Maximum Marks: 25

S. No.	Contents	Maximum marks	Marks obtained
1.	Patient's history	03	
2.	Assessment	10	
3.	Complication and prognosis	06	
4.	Health teaching	03	
5.	Conclusion	03	
	Total	**25**	

Remarks:

Signature of Student

Signature of Supervisor

Patient's Identification Data

- Name   :
- Age   :
- Sex   :
- Marital status   :
- Hospital registration no.   :
- Ward/bed no.   :
- Address   :
- Tel. no.   :
- Religion   :
- Education   :
- Date of admission   :
- Date of discharge   :
- Diagnosis   :
- Operation   :
- Date of operation   :
- Name of the doctor   :
- Occupation   :
- Monthly family income (₹)   :
- Nursing alert   :
- Sensitivity/allergy/precaution   :
- Weight   :
- Height   :

Informant

Information's relevant or not.

NEUROLOGICAL EXAMINATION

Assessing Consciousness and Cognition

- Level of consciousness: Alert/lethargic/stuporous/semicomatose/comatose

- Emotional state: Anxious/calm/angry cooperative/fearful/restless/withdrawn

- Vital signs:

  - Temp:

  - Pulse:

  - BP:

  - Respiration:

  - SpO_2:

  - Pain score: Pain scale

Time						
Score						

- Glasgow coma scale:

Action	Response	Score
Eyes open	• Spontaneously • To speech • To pain • None	4 3 2 1
Verbal response	• Oriented • Confused • Inappropriate words • Incomprehensible sound • None	5 4 3 2 1
Motor response	• Obeys commands • Movement to localized pain • Withdrawn the pain • Abnormal flexion • Abnormal extension • None	6 5 4 3 2 1
Total score = 15		Total =
<15 = Moderate risk, <9 = High-risk, 13–15= Really alert, <8 = Unconscious, <3 = Coma		

Mental Status Examinations

- General appearance
  - Body build: Thin/obese/normal
  - Posture: Normal (erect and upright)/scoliosis/lordosis kyphosis
  - Hygiene and grooming: Clean unclean/self-care deficit
- Communication: Relevant/irrelevant/slurred speech/confusion incomprehensible sound/aphasia
- Mood and effect: Appropriate/agitation/anger/depression/euphoria
- Thought content: Normal/illusions/hallucination/delusions
- Cognition function:
  - Orientation: Oriented to time, place, person not oriented
  - Memory: Intact immediate, recent, and remote memory/abnormally in anyone
  - Judgment: Normal/abnormal
  - Insight: Present/absent

Assessing Cranial Nerve Function

- Olfactory (sensory)
  - Sense of smell: Present/absent
- Optic (sensory)
  - Inspection of eye: Normal/inflammation/cataract/any abnormalities
  - Visual acuity test (by Snellen chart): Normal/abnormal
  - Visual field test/confrontation test: Normal/abnormal
  - Color detection: Present/absent
  - Fundoscopy reveals: Normal/abnormal
- Oculomotor, trochlear and abducens (motor)
  - Pupillary reaction to light: Reacting/not reacting
  - Pupillary size: Equal/unequal
  - Eye movement in six directions: Normal/abnormal
  - Convergence and accommodation: Normal/abnormal
  - Nystagmus: Present/absent
  - Diplopia: Present/absent
- Trigeminal (mixed)
  - Sensory
    - Facial sensory response: Present/absent
  - Motor
    - Mandibular strength test: Adequate hypotonia
    - Corneal reflex: Present/absent
- Facial (mixed)
  - Motor (facial expression): Normal/hypotonia
  - Sensory (taste sensation): Present/absent

- Vestibulocochlear
  - Auditory: Normal/abnormal
- Glossopharyngeal and vagus (mixed)
  - Gas reflex: Present/absent
  - Swallowing reflex
  - Position and movement of uvula and palate: Normal position deviation
  - Sensation of taste: Present/absent
- Spinal accessory (motor)
  - Sternocleidomastoid muscle strength: Normal/hypotonia
  - Elevation of shoulders: Adequate strength weakness
  - Turning of head: Adequate/inadequate
- Hypoglossal (motor)
  - Tongue movement: Normal/abnormal

Motor System Assessment

- Muscle size: Normal/abnormal
- Assessing muscle strength
  - Upper extremities
    - Neck: Normal/good/fair/poor/trace/no response
    - Shoulder (trapezius): Normal/good/fair/poor/trace/no response
    - Biceps: Normal/good/fair/poor/trace/no response
    - Triceps: Normal/good/fair/poor/trace/no response
  - Lower extremities
    - Quadriceps: Normal/good/fair/poor/trace/no response
    - Gastroenemius: Normal/good/fair/poor/trace/no response

Muscle strength maneuver result		
Parameter	**Description**	**Score**
Normal (100%)	Very strong with range of motion unimpaired against gravity and against full resistance.	5
Good (75%)	Adequate strength to complete range of motion against gravity and against a mild to moderate level of resistance.	4
Fair (50%)	Only enough strength to complete against gravity but not against any additional resistance.	3
Poor (25%)	Very weak with inability to complete range of motion unless gravity eliminated by external assistance.	2
Trace (10%)	A weak muscle contraction when muscle palpated but no movement.	1
No response (0%)	Complete paralysis.	0

- Muscle tone: Normal/hypotonia/hypertonia
- Muscle coordination: Normal/abnormal
- Gait: Normal/abnormal
- Movements of all joints: Present/absent
- Deformities: Present/absent
- Abnormal movements (tics/tremor/chorea/athetosis/myoclonus): Present/absent

Assessing Sensory Function

- Pain sensation: Present/absent
- Temperature sensation: Present/absent
- Touch sensation: Present/absent
- Vibration sensation: Present/absent
- Position sense: Present/absent
- Discrimination
    - Astereognosis or tactile agnosia: Present/absent
    - Visual agnosia: Present/absent

Cerebellar Functioning

- Gait: Normal/hemiparetic gait/ataxic gait/steppage gait
- Posture: Normal (erect and upright)/scoliosis lordosis/kyphosis
- Romberg's test: Normal/abnormal
- Nose to finger test: Normal/abnormal
- Finger to finger test: Normal/abnormal
- Heel to shin test: Normal/abnormal

Assessing Reflexes

- Deep tendon reflexes:
    - Upper extremities
        - Biceps: Present (flexion of arm at elbow)/partially/absent
        - Triceps: Present (extension at elbow)/partially/absent
        - Brachioradialis: Present (extension at elbow)/partially/absent
    - Lower extremities
        - Patellar reflex: Present (extension of lower leg at knee)/partially/absent
        - Achilles reflex: Present (planter flexion of foot)/partially/absent
- Superficial reflexes:
    - Abnormal reflex: Present/absent
    - Corneal reflex: Present/absent
    - Gag reflex: Present/absent
    - Plantar reflex: Present/absent
- Pathological reflex
    - Babinski reflex: Planter flexion (toes contract and draw together)/toes fan out and draw back

Complications and Prognosis

Health Teaching

Summary and Conclusion

Case Study

▌ EVALUATION CRITERIA FOR NURSING CASE STUDY

Maximum Marks: 100

S. No.	Contents	Maximum marks	Marks obtained
1.	Patient's history	04	
2.	Physical examination	04	
3.	Anatomy and physiology	05	
4.	Incidence and etiology	05	
5.	Pathophysiology	05	
6.	Clinical manifestations	06	
7.	Investigations	04	
8.	Complication and prognosis	05	
9.	Management: Medical and surgical	12	
10.	Drug study	10	
11.	Nursing care plan	15	
12.	Nurses' notes	08	
13.	Health education	06	
14.	Discharge planning	05	
15.	Conclusion and research evidence	03	
16.	Bibliography	03	
	Total	**100**	

Remarks:

Signature of Student   **Signature of Supervisor**

Introduction

Purposes of the Study

Objectives of the Study

Duration of the Study

Objectives of the Study

Patient's Identification Data

- Name :
- Age :
- Sex :
- Marital status :
- Hospital registration no. :
- Ward/bed no. :
- Address :
- Tel. no. :
- Religion :
- Education :
- Date of admission :
- Date of discharge :
- Diagnosis :
- Operation :
- Date of operation :
- Name of the doctor :
- Occupation :
- Monthly family income (₹) :
- Nursing alert :
- Sensitivity/allergy/precaution :
- Weight :
- Height :

Informant

Information's relevant or not.

Chief Complaints with Duration

History of Present Illness

History of Past Medical Illness: Illness/medications/any restrictions.

History of Past Surgical Illness: Illness/medications/any restrictions.

Obstetrical History

Family History

S. No.	Name of family member	Age and sex	Relationship with patient	Occupation	Health status/ history of significant illness	Health habits

Family Tree

Socioeconomic History

- Occupation and social relationship:
- Monthly family income (₹):
- Health facility near home:
  - Type:
    - Hospital
    - Health center
    - Any other: If any other (specify)
  - Distance: ___________ kms.
  - Transportation facility:
    - Yes
    - No
  - Housing: Type
    - Kutcha
    - Pucca
  - No. of rooms:
  - Toilet: Indian/western/temporary/open
  - Electricity: Yes/No
  - Drinking water source: Tap/well/pond/river/hand/pump

Dietary History

Health Habits: Functional Health Pattern

- Health perception/health management:

- Nutritional/metabolic:

- Elimination:

- Activity/exercise:

- Sleep/rest:

- Self-perception/self-concept:

- Role relationship:

- Sexuality/reproductive:

- Coping/stress–tolerance:

- Value/belief:

- Other comments/data:

Physical Examination

General Appearance

Height

Weight

Vital Signs

S. No.	Vital signs	Patient value	Normal value	Remarks
1.	Temperature			
2.	Pulse			
3.	Respiration			
4.	Blood pressure			

Head

- Scalp:
- Face:
- Sinus:
- Nodes:

Eyes

- Ocular movement:
- Pupils:
- Sclera:
- Cornea:

Ears

- External structures:
- Hearing:

Nose

- External structure:
- Septum:
- Mucous membrane:
- Patency:
- Olfactory sense:

Mouth

- Buccal mucosa:
- Gums:
- Teeth:
- Palates and uvula:
- Tonsillar area:
- Voice breath:

Neck

- Muscles:
- Trachea:
- Thyroid:
- Nodes:
- Vein distension:

Thorax

- Chest shape:
- Respiratory rate:
- Type of respiration:
- Thoracic expansion:
- Palpation:
- Percussion:
- Breath sounds:

Cardiovascular System

- Precordium: Inspection:
- Palpation:
- Auscultation:
- Apical rate and rhythm:

Central and Peripheral Vessels

- Carotid arteries:
- Peripheral pulses: Brachial:
- Radial:
- Femoral:
- Popliteal:

- Dorsal pedal:
- Posterior tibial:
- Capillary refill:

Abdomen

- Inspection:
- Auscultation:
- Percussion:
- Palpation:

Musculoskeletal System

- Gait:
- Upper extremities:
- Lower extremities:
- Muscle strength:
- Joints:
- Range of motion:
- Spine:

Nervous System

- Mental status:
  - Language:
  - Orientation:
  - Memory attention span:
- Level of consciousness (GCS):
- Cranial nerves:
- Deep tendon reflex:
- Gross and fine motor function of UE and LE:
- Sensory function:
  - Light touch:
  - Pain:
  - Temperature:
- Position:

Genitalia and Rectal Examination

- Inspection:
- Palpation:

Comparison of the Patient's Disease with Book Picture

- Definition

- Anatomy and physiology

- Incidence

- Etiology

Book picture	Patient picture

- Pathophysiology

- Signs and symptoms

- Diagnosis provisional and final

Book picture	Patient picture

Investigations

Date	Investigations done	Normal value	Patient value	Inference

Management: Medical or Surgical

Drug Study

S. No.	Drug trade name	Pharmacological name	Dose and frequency	Route	Action	Side effects and drug interaction	Nurses responsibility

Nursing Care Plan

Nursing assessment: Subjective and objective data	Nursing diagnosis	Goals	Nursing intervention		Rationale	Evaluation
			Planned	Implemented		

Nurses' Notes

Time	Medication	Diet/nutrition	Observation/intervention/evaluation	Signature

Complications and Prognosis

Health Teaching

Summary and Conclusion

Bibliography

Case Presentation

▌EVALUATION CRITERIA FOR NURSING CASE PRESENTATION

Maximum Marks: 100

S. No.	Contents	Maximum marks	Marks obtained
1.	Assessment	10	
2.	Co-relation with patient and book	15	
3.	Drug study	06	
4.	Nursing care plan	25	
5.	Nurses' notes	05	
6.	Health education	06	
7.	Use of AV aids	08	
8.	Physical arrangement	05	
9.	Group participation	10	
10.	Effectiveness of presentation	05	
11.	Bibliography	05	
	Total	**100**	

Remarks:

Signature of Student   **Signature of Supervisor**

Patient's Identification Data

- Name   :
- Age   :
- Sex   :
- Marital status   :
- Hospital registration no.   :
- Ward/bed no.   :
- Address   :
- Tel. no.   :
- Religion   :
- Education   :
- Date of admission   :
- Date of discharge   :
- Diagnosis   :
- Operation   :
- Date of operation   :
- Name of the doctor   :
- Occupation   :
- Monthly family income (₹)   :
- Nursing alert   :
- Sensitivity/allergy/precaution   :
- Weight   :
- Height   :

Informant

Information's relevant or not.

Chief Complaints with Duration

History of Present Illness

History of Past Medical Illness: Illness/medications/any restrictions.

History of Past Surgical Illness: Illness/medications/any restrictions.

Obstetrical History

Family History

S. No.	Name of family member	Age and sex	Relationship with patient	Occupation	Health status/ history of significant illness	Health habits

Family Tree

Socioeconomic History

- Occupation and social relationship:
- Monthly family income (₹):
- Health facility near home:
  - Type:
    - Hospital
    - Health center
    - Any other: If any other (specify)
  - Distance: __________ kms.
  - Transportation facility:
    - Yes
    - No
  - Housing: Type
    - Kutcha
    - Pucca
  - No. of rooms:
  - Toilet: Indian/western/temporary/open
  - Electricity: Yes/No
  - Drinking water source: Tap/well/pond/river/hand/pump

Dietary History

Health Habits: Functional Health Pattern

- Health perception/health management:

- Nutritional/metabolic:

- Elimination:

- Activity/exercise:

- Sleep/rest:

- Self-perception/self-concept:

- Role relationship:

- Sexuality/reproductive:

- Coping/stress–tolerance:

- Value/belief:

- Other comments/data:

Physical Examination

General Appearance

Height

Weight

Vital Signs

S. No.	Vital signs	Patient value	Normal value	Remarks
1.	Temperature			
2.	Pulse			
3.	Respiration			
4.	Blood pressure			

Head

- Scalp:
- Face:
- Sinus:
- Nodes:

Eyes

- Ocular movement:
- Pupils:
- Sclera:
- Cornea:

Ears

- External structures:
- Hearing:

Nose

- External structure:
- Septum:
- Mucous membrane:
- Patency:
- Olfactory sense:

Mouth

- Buccal mucosa:
- Gums:
- Teeth:
- Palates and uvula:
- Tonsillar area:
- Voice breath:

Neck

- Muscles:
- Trachea:
- Thyroid:
- Nodes:
- Vein distension:

Thorax

- Chest shape:
- Respiratory rate:
- Type of respiration:
- Thoracic expansion:
- Palpation:
- Percussion:
- Breath sounds:

Cardiovascular System

- Precordium—Inspection:
- Palpation:
- Auscultation:
- Apical rate and rhythm:

Central and Peripheral Vessels

- Carotid arteries:
- Peripheral pulses—Brachial:
- Radial:
- Femoral:
- Popliteal:
- Dorsal pedal:
- Posterior tibial:
- Capillary refill:

Abdomen

- Inspection:

- Auscultation:

- Percussion:

- Palpation:

Musculoskeletal System

- Gait:

- Upper extremities:

- Lower extremities:

- Muscle strength:

- Joints:

- Range of motion:

- Spine:

Nervous System

- Mental status:

    - Language:

    - Orientation:

    - Memory attention span:

- Level of consciousness (GCS):

- Cranial nerves:

- Deep tendon reflex:

- Gross and fine motor function of UE and LE:

- Sensory function:

    - Light touch:

    - Pain:

    - Temperature:

- Position:

Genitalia and Rectal Examination

- Inspection:

- Palpation:

Comparison of the Patient's Disease with Book Picture

- Anatomy and physiology

- Incidence

- Etiology

S. No.	Book picture	Patient picture

- Pathophysiology

- Clinical manifestations

S. No.	Book picture	Patient picture

- Diagnosis provisional and final

S. No.	Book picture	Patient picture

Investigations

Date	Investigations done	Normal value	Patient value	Inference

Management: Medical or Surgical

Drug Study

S. No.	Drug trade name	Pharmacological name	Dose and frequency	Route	Action	Side effects and drug interaction	Nurses responsibility

Drug Study

Nursing Care Plan

Nursing assessment: Subjective and objective data	Nursing diagnosis	Goals	Nursing intervention		Rationale	Evaluation
			Planned	Implemented		

Nurses' Notes

Time	Medication	Diet/nutrition	Observation/intervention/evaluation	Signature

Complications and Prognosis

Health Teaching

Discharge Planning/Notes

Summary and Conclusion

Bibliography

Drug Presentation

EVALUATION CRITERIA FOR DRUG PRESENTATION

Maximum Marks: 25

S. No.	Contents	Maximum marks	Marks obtained
1.	Name of drug	02	
2.	Dose, time and route	02	
3.	Action	03	
4.	Indication	03	
5.	Contraindication	03	
6.	Side-effects	03	
7.	Nursing responsibilities	07	
8.	Conclusion	02	
	Total	**25**	

Remarks:

Signature of Student   **Signature of Supervisor**

Introduction

Drug Name and Classification

Indication

Mechanism of Action

Dosage and Administration

Side Effects and Adverse Reactions

Contraindication and Precautions

Drug Interactions

Patient Education

Nursing Responsibility

Conclusion

Bibliography

Nursing Management of Patients with Immunological Disorders

- ☑ Immune System Assessment
- ☑ Health Teaching
- ☑ Nutritional Assessment
- ☑ Nursing Care Plan

Immune System Assessment

■ EVALUATION CRITERIA FOR IMMUNE SYSTEM ASSESSMENT

Maximum Marks: 25

S. No.	Contents	Maximum marks	Marks obtained
1.	Patient's history	03	
2.	Assessment	10	
3.	Complication and prognosis	06	
4.	Health teaching	03	
5.	Conclusion	03	
	Total	**25**	

Remarks:

Signature of Student   **Signature of Supervisor**

Patient's Identification Data

- Name   :
- Age   :
- Sex   :
- Marital status   :
- Hospital registration no.   :
- Ward/bed no.   :
- Address   :
- Tel. no.   :
- Religion   :
- Education   :
- Date of admission   :
- Date of discharge   :
- Diagnosis   :
- Operation   :
- Date of operation   :
- Name of the doctor   :
- Occupation   :
- Monthly family income (₹)   :
- Nursing alert   :
- Sensitivity/allergy/precaution   :
- Weight   :
- Height   :

Informant

Information's relevant or not.

History Collection

- Past and present condition:

- Infection and immunization:

- Nutrition:

Disorder and Disease

- Autoimmune disorder:

- Neoplastic disease:

- Chronic illness and surgery:

- Special problems (burn):

Medication and Blood Transfusion

Lifestyle Factor

Physical Examination

Skin and Mucous Membrane

- Lesions:

- Dermatitis:

- Purpura:

- Urticarial:

- Inflammation:

- Discharges:

- Sign of infection:

- Lymph node enlargement:

Diagnostic Evaluation

- Blood test:

- Skin test:

- Bone marrow biopsy:

- Humoral immunity test:

- Cellular immunity test:

- Delayed hypersensitivity test:

Complications and Prognosis

Health Teaching

Summary and Conclusion

Health Teaching

■ EVALUATION CRITERIA FOR HEALTH TEACHING

- Name of the institution:

- Name of the student:

- Language:

- Topic:

- Audience:

- Ward/field:

- Name of the supervisor/teacher: Date:

S. No.	Criteria	Marks allotted	Marks obtained
	Content		
1.	Lesson planning	05	
2.	Appropriateness, relevancy and adequacy of content	08	
3.	Organization	04	
4.	Up to date and evidence-based	03	
	Presentation		
1.	Physical arrangement	03	
2	Communication skill	05	
3.	Confidence	03	
4.	Group involvement	03	
	AV aids		
1.	Selection and preparation	04	
2.	Effective use of AV aids	03	
	Other		
1.	Time management	03	
2.	Acceptance of guidance	03	
3.	Reference	03	
	Total	**50**	

Signature of Student   **Signature of Supervisor**

Health Education

Topic Selected

- Name of the student teacher :
- Name of the supervisor :
- Venue :
- Date :
- Time :
- Group :
- Previous knowledge of the group :
- AV aids used :
- General objectives:

- Specific objectives:

Lesson Plan for Health Talk

S. No.	Time	Specific objectives	Contents	Teaching-learning activities	AV aids	Evaluation

Nutritional Assessment

EVALUATION CRITERIA FOR NUTRITIONAL ASSESSMENT

Maximum Marks: 25

S. No.	Contents	Maximum marks	Marks obtained
1.	Patient's history	03	
2.	Assessment	10	
3.	Complication and prognosis	06	
4.	Health teaching	03	
5.	Conclusion	03	
	Total	**25**	

Remarks:

Signature of Student　　　　　　　　　　　　　　　　　　　　**Signature of Supervisor**

Patient's Identification Data

- Name :

- Age :

- Sex :

- Marital status :

- Hospital registration no. :

- Ward/bed no. :

- Address :

- Telephone no. :

- Religion :

- Education :

- Date of admission :

- Date of discharge :

- Diagnosis :

- Operation :

- Date of operation :

- Name of the doctor :

- Occupation :

- Monthly family income (₹) :

- Nursing alert :

- Sensitivity/allergy/precaution :

Anthropometric Measurements

- Height:

- Weight:

- BMI:

Dietary History

- Meal patterns (e.g., number of meals, snacks)

- Food preferences and dislikes

- Special dietary restrictions or considerations (e.g., allergies, cultural/religious restrictions)

- Recent changes in appetite or dietary intake

- Assess for any signs of malnutrition or nutritional deficiencies

Nutritional Assessment

- Body composition (e.g., muscle mass, fat distribution)

- Signs of malnutrition (e.g., dry skin, brittle hair, muscle wasting)

- Nutrient deficiencies (e.g., iron deficiency, vitamin D deficiency)

- Energy and macronutrient needs

- Micronutrient needs

Vitamins and Minerals

- Vitamin A, C, D, E, K

- B vitamins (e.g., B_{12}, folate)

- Calcium, iron, zinc, magnesium

Fluid and Hydration Status

Complications and Prognosis

Health Teaching

Summary and Conclusion

Nursing Care Plan

EVALUATION CRITERIA FOR NURSING CARE PLAN

Maximum Marks: 25

S. No.	Contents	Maximum marks	Allotted marks
1.	Patient's history	02	
2.	Physical examination	02	
3.	Investigations	01	
4.	Drug study	02	
5.	Nursing care plan • Assessment • Nursing diagnosis • Goals • Expected outcome • Nursing intervention • Rationale • Evaluation	02 02 02 01 01 03 01	
6.	Nurses' notes	03	
7.	Health education	02	
8.	Bibliography	01	
	Total	**25**	

Remarks:

Signature of Student   **Signature of Supervisor**

Patient's Identification Data

- Name :
- Age :
- Sex :
- Marital status :
- Hospital registration no. :
- Ward/bed no. :
- Address :
- Tel. no. :
- Religion :
- Education :
- Date of admission :
- Date of discharge :
- Diagnosis :
- Operation :
- Date of operation :
- Name of the doctor :
- Occupation :
- Monthly family income (₹) :
- Nursing alert :
- Sensitivity/allergy/precaution :
- Weight :
- Height :

Informant

Information's relevant or not.

Chief Complaints with Duration

History of Present Illness

History of Past Medical Illness: Illness/medications/any restrictions.

History of Past Surgical Illness: Illness/medications/any restrictions.

Obstetrical History

Family History

S. No.	Name of family member	Age and sex	Relationship with patient	Occupation	Health status/ history of significant illness	Health habits

Family Tree

Socioeconomic History

- Occupation and social relationship:
- Monthly family income (₹):
- Health facility near home:
    - Type:
        - Hospital
        - Health center
        - Any other: If any other (specify)
    - Distance: ___________ kms.
    - Transportation facility:
        - Yes
        - No
    - Housing: Type
        - Kutcha
        - Pucca
    - No. of rooms:
    - Toilet: Indian/western/temporary/open
    - Electricity: Yes/No
    - Drinking water source: Tap/well/pond/river/hand/pump

Dietary History

Health Habits: Functional Health Pattern

- Health perception/health management:

- Nutritional/metabolic:

- Elimination:

- Activity/exercise:

- Sleep/rest:

- Self-perception/self-concept:

- Role relationship:

- Sexuality/reproductive:

- Coping/stress–tolerance:

- Value/belief:

- Other comments/data:

Physical Examination

General Appearance

Height

Weight

Vital Signs

S. No.	Vital signs	Patient value	Normal value	Remarks
1.	Temperature			
2.	Pulse			
3.	Respiration			
4.	Blood pressure			

Head

- Scalp:
- Face:
- Sinus:
- Nodes:

Eyes

- Ocular movement:
- Pupils:
- Sclera:
- Cornea:

Ears

- External structures:
- Hearing:

Nose

- External structure:
- Septum:
- Mucous membrane:
- Patency:
- Olfactory sense:

Mouth

- Buccal mucosa:
- Gums:
- Teeth:
- Palates and uvula:
- Tonsillar area:
- Voice breath:

Neck

- Muscles:
- Trachea:
- Thyroid:
- Nodes:
- Vein distension:

Thorax

- Chest shape:
- Respiratory rate:
- Type of respiration:
- Thoracic expansion:
- Palpation:
- Percussion:
- Breath sounds:

Cardiovascular System

- Precordium: Inspection:
- Palpation:
- Auscultation:
- Apical rate and rhythm:

Central and Peripheral Vessels

- Carotid arteries:
- Peripheral pulses: Brachial:
- Radial:
- Femoral:
- Popliteal:
- Dorsal pedal:
- Posterior tibial:
- Capillary refill:

Abdomen

- Inspection:
- Auscultation:
- Percussion:
- Palpation:

Musculoskeletal System

- Gait:
- Upper extremities:
- Lower extremities:
- Muscle strength:
- Joints:
- Range of motion:
- Spine

Nervous System

- Mental status:
  - Language:
  - Orientation:
  - Memory attention span:
- Level of consciousness (GCS):
- Cranial nerves:
- Deep tendon reflex:
- Gross and fine motor function of UE and LE:
- Sensory function:
  - Light touch:
  - Pain:
  - Temperature:
- Position:

Genitalia and Rectal Examination

- Inspection:
- Palpation:

Investigations

Date	Investigations done	Normal value	Patient value	Inference

Management: Medical or Surgical

Drug Study

S. No.	Drug trade name	Pharmacological name	Dose and frequency	Route	Action	Side effects and drug interaction	Nurses responsibility

Nursing Care Plan

Nursing assessment: Subjective and objective data	Nursing diagnosis	Goals	Nursing intervention		Rationale	Evaluation
			Planned	Implemented		

Nurses' Notes

Time	Medication	Diet/nutrition	Observation/ intervention/evaluation	Signature

Complications and Prognosis

Health Teaching

Discharge Planning/Notes

Summary and Conclusion Including Research Evidence

Bibliography

Nursing Management of Patients with Disorder of Oncological Conditions

- ☑ Case Study
- ☑ Case Presentation
- ☑ Health Teaching
- ☑ Educational Visits

Case Study

■ EVALUATION CRITERIA FOR NURSING CASE STUDY

Maximum Marks: 100

S. No.	Contents	Maximum marks	Marks obtained
1.	Patient's history	04	
2.	Physical examination	04	
3.	Anatomy and physiology	05	
4.	Incidence and etiology	05	
5.	Pathophysiology	05	
6.	Clinical manifestations	06	
7.	Investigations	04	
8.	Complication and prognosis	05	
9.	Management: Medical and surgical	12	
10.	Drug study	10	
11.	Nursing care plan	15	
12.	Nurses' notes	08	
13.	Health education	06	
14.	Discharge planning	05	
15.	Conclusion and research evidence	03	
16.	Bibliography	03	
	Total	**100**	

Remarks:

Signature of Student   **Signature of Supervisor**

Introduction

Purposes of the Study

Objectives of the Study

Duration of the Study

Patient's Identification Data

- Name :
- Age :
- Sex :
- Marital status :
- Hospital registration no. :
- Ward/bed no. :
- Address :
- Tel. no. :
- Religion :
- Education :
- Date of admission :
- Date of discharge :
- Diagnosis :
- Operation :
- Date of operation :
- Name of the doctor :
- Occupation :
- Monthly family income (₹) :
- Nursing alert :
- Sensitivity/allergy/precaution :
- Weight :
- Height :

Informant

Information's relevant or not.

Chief Complaints with Duration

History of Present Illness

History of Past Medical Illness: Illness/medications/any restrictions.

History of Past Surgical Illness: Illness/medications/any restrictions.

Obstetrical History

Family History

S. No.	Name of family member	Age and sex	Relationship with patient	Occupation	Health status/ history of significant illness	Health habits

Family Tree

Socioeconomic History

- Occupation and social relationship:
- Monthly family income (₹):
- Health facility near home:
  - Type:
    - Hospital
    - Health center
    - Any other: If any other (specify)
  - Distance: _________ kms.
  - Transportation facility:
    - Yes
    - No
  - Housing: Type
    - Kutcha
    - Pucca
  - No. of rooms:
  - Toilet: Indian/western/temporary/open
  - Electricity: Yes/No
  - Drinking water source: Tap/well/pond/river/hand/pump

Dietary History

Health Habits: Functional Health Pattern

- Health perception/health management:

- Nutritional/metabolic:

- Elimination:

- Activity/exercise:

- Sleep/rest:

- Self-perception/self-concept:

- Role relationship:

- Sexuality/reproductive:

- Coping/stress–tolerance:

- Value/belief:

- Other comments/data:

Physical Examination

General Appearance

Height

Weight

Vital Signs

S. No.	Vital signs	Patient value	Normal value	Remarks
1.	Temperature			
2.	Pulse			
3.	Respiration			
4.	Blood pressure			

Head

- Scalp:
- Face:
- Sinus:
- Nodes:

Eyes

- Ocular movement:
- Pupils:
- Sclera:
- Cornea:

Ears

- External structures:
- Hearing:

Nose

- External structure:
- Septum:
- Mucous membrane:
- Patency:
- Olfactory sense:

Mouth

- Buccal mucosa:
- Gums:
- Teeth:
- Palates and uvula:
- Tonsillar area:
- Voice breath:

Neck

- Muscles:
- Trachea:
- Thyroid:
- Nodes:
- Vein distension:

Thorax

- Chest shape:
- Respiratory rate:
- Type of respiration:
- Thoracic expansion:
- Palpation:
- Percussion:
- Breath sounds:

Cardiovascular System

- Precordium: Inspection:
- Palpation:
- Auscultation:
- Apical rate and rhythm:

Central and Peripheral Vessels

- Carotid arteries:
- Peripheral pulses: Brachial:
- Radial:
- Femoral:
- Popliteal:
- Dorsal pedal:
- Posterior tibial:
- Capillary refill:

Abdomen

- Inspection:
- Auscultation:
- Percussion:
- Palpation:

Musculoskeletal System

- Gait:
- Upper extremities:
- Lower extremities:
- Muscle strength:
- Joints:
- Range of motion:
- Spine:

Nervous System

- Mental status:
    - Language:
    - Orientation:
    - Memory attention span:
- Level of consciousness (GCS):
- Cranial nerves:
- Deep tendon reflex:
- Gross and fine motor function of UE and LE:
- Sensory function:
    - Light touch:
    - Pain:
    - Temperature:
- Position:

Genitalia and Rectal Examination

- Inspection:
- Palpation:

Comparison of the Patient's Disease with Book Picture

- Definition

- Anatomy and physiology

- Incidence

- Etiology

Book picture	Patient picture

- Pathophysiology

- Signs and symptoms

- Diagnosis provisional and final

Book picture	Patient picture

Investigations

Date	Investigations done	Normal value	Patient value	Inference

Management: Medical or Surgical

Drug Study

S. No.	Drug trade name	Pharmacological name	Dose and frequency	Route	Action	Side effects and drug interaction	Nurses responsibility

Nursing Care Plan

Nursing assessment: Subjective and objective data	Nursing diagnosis	Goals	Nursing intervention		Rationale	Evaluation
			Planned	Implemented		

Nurses' Notes

Time	Medication	Diet/nutrition	Observation/ intervention/evaluation	Signature

Complications and Prognosis

Health Teaching

Summary and Conclusion

Bibliography

Case Presentation

▌ EVALUATION CRITERIA FOR NURSING CASE PRESENTATION

Maximum Marks: 100

S. No.	Contents	Maximum marks	Marks obtained
1.	Assessment	10	
2.	Co-relation with patient and book	15	
3.	Drug study	06	
4.	Nursing care plan	25	
5.	Nurses' notes	05	
6.	Health education	06	
7.	Use of AV aids	08	
8.	Physical arrangement	05	
9.	Group participation	10	
10.	Effectiveness of presentation	05	
11.	Bibliography	05	
	Total	**100**	

Remarks:

Signature of Student   **Signature of Supervisor**

Patient's Identification Data

- Name :
- Age :
- Sex :
- Marital status :
- Hospital registration no. :
- Ward/bed no. :
- Address :
- Tel. no. :
- Religion :
- Education :
- Date of admission :
- Date of discharge :
- Diagnosis :
- Operation :
- Date of operation :
- Name of the doctor :
- Occupation :
- Monthly family income (₹) :
- Nursing alert :
- Sensitivity/allergy/precaution :
- Weight :
- Height :

Informant

Information's relevant or not.

Chief Complaints with Duration

History of Present Illness

History of Past Medical Illness: Illness/medications/any restrictions.

History of Past Surgical Illness: Illness/medications/any restrictions.

Obstetrical History

Family History

S. No.	Name of family member	Age and sex	Relationship with patient	Occupation	Health status/ history of significant illness	Health habits

Family Tree

Socioeconomic History

- Occupation and social relationship:
- Monthly family income (₹):
- Health facility near home:
  - Type:
    - Hospital
    - Health center
    - Any other: If any other (specify)
  - Distance: __________ kms.
  - Transportation facility:
    - Yes
    - No
  - Housing: Type
    - Kutcha
    - Pucca
  - No. of rooms:
  - Toilet: Indian/western/temporary/open
  - Electricity: Yes/No
  - Drinking water source: Tap/well/pond/river/hand/pump

Dietary History

Health Habits: Functional Health Pattern

- Health perception/health management:

- Nutritional/metabolic:

- Elimination:

- Activity/exercise:

- Sleep/rest:

- Self-perception/self-concept:

- Role relationship:

- Sexuality/reproductive:

- Coping/stress–tolerance:

- Value/belief:

- Other comments/data:

Physical Examination

General Appearance

Height

Weight

Vital Signs

S. No.	Vital signs	Patient value	Normal value	Remarks
1.	Temperature			
2.	Pulse			
3.	Respiration			
4.	Blood pressure			

Head

- Scalp:
- Face:
- Sinus:
- Nodes:

Eyes

- Ocular movement:
- Pupils:
- Sclera:
- Cornea:

Ears

- External structures:
- Hearing:

Nose

- External structure:
- Septum:
- Mucous membrane:
- Patency:
- Olfactory sense:

Mouth

- Buccal mucosa:
- Gums:
- Teeth:
- Palates and uvula:
- Tonsillar area:
- Voice breath:

Neck

- Muscles:
- Trachea:
- Thyroid:
- Nodes:
- Vein distension:

Thorax

- Chest shape:
- Respiratory rate:
- Type of respiration:
- Thoracic expansion:
- Palpation:
- Percussion:
- Breath sounds:

Cardiovascular System

- Precordium: Inspection:
- Palpation:
- Auscultation:
- Apical rate and rhythm:

Central and Peripheral Vessels

- Carotid arteries:
- Peripheral pulses: Brachial:
- Radial:
- Femoral:
- Popliteal:
- Dorsal pedal:
- Posterior tibial:
- Capillary refill:

Abdomen

- Inspection:
- Auscultation:
- Percussion:
- Palpation:

Musculoskeletal System

- Gait:
- Upper extremities:
- Lower extremities:
- Muscle strength:
- Joints:
- Range of motion:
- Spine:

Nervous System

- Mental status:
  - Language:
  - Orientation:
  - Memory attention span:
- Level of consciousness (GCS):
- Cranial nerves:
- Deep tendon reflex:
- Gross and fine motor function of UE and LE:
- Sensory function:
  - Light touch:
  - Pain:
  - Temperature:
- Position:

Genitalia and Rectal Examination

- Inspection:
- Palpation:

Comparison of the Patient's Disease with Book Picture

- Anatomy and physiology

- Incidence

- Etiology

S. No.	Book picture	Patient picture

- Pathophysiology

- Clinical manifestations

S. No.	Book picture	Patient picture

- Diagnosis provisional and final

S. No.	Book picture	Patient picture

Investigations

Date	Investigations done	Normal value	Patient value	Inference

Management: Medical or Surgical

Drug Study

S. No.	Drug trade name	Pharmacological name	Dose and frequency	Route	Action	Side effects and drug interaction	Nurses responsibility

Nursing Care Plan

Nursing assessment: Subjective and objective data	Nursing diagnosis	Goals	Nursing intervention		Rationale	Evaluation
			Planned	Implemented		

Nurses' Notes

Time	Medication	Diet/nutrition	Observation/ intervention/evaluation	Signature

Complications and Prognosis

Health Teaching

Discharge Planning/Notes

Summary and Conclusion

Bibliography

Health Teaching

▌ EVALUATION CRITERIA FOR HEALTH TEACHING

- Name of the institution   :
- Name of the student   :
- Language   :
- Topic   :
- Audience   :
- Ward/field   :
- Name of the supervisor/teacher   :   Date:

S. No.	Criteria	Marks allotted	Marks obtained
	Content		
1.	Lesson planning	05	
2.	Appropriateness, relevancy and adequacy of content	08	
3.	Organization	04	
4.	Up to date and evidence based	03	
	Presentation		
1.	Physical arrangement	03	
2.	Communication skill	05	
3.	Confidence	03	
4.	Group involvement	03	
	AV aids		
1.	Selection and preparation	04	
2.	Effective use of AV aids	03	
	Other		
1.	Time management	03	
2.	Acceptance of guidance	03	
3.	Reference	03	
	Total	**50**	

Signature of Student   **Signature of Supervisor**

Health Education

Topic Selected

- Name of the student teacher   :
- Name of the supervisor   :
- Venue   :
- Date   :
- Time   :
- Group   :
- Previous knowledge of the group   :
- AV aids used   :
- General objectives:

- Specific objectives:

Lesson Plan for Health Talk

S. No.	Time	Specific objectives	Contents	Teaching-learning activities	AV Aids	Evaluation

Educational Visits

EVALUATION PROFORMA FOR EDUCATIONAL VISIT

Maximum Marks: 10

S. No.	Contents	Maximum marks	Marks obtained
1.	Introduction	1	
2.	Objectives	1	
3.	Organization pattern	1	
4.	Staffing pattern	1	
5.	Physical set-up	1	
6.	Description	3	
7.	Submission of report on time	1	
8.	Conclusion	1	
	Total	**10**	

Remarks:

Signature of Student   **Signature of Supervisor**

Palliative Care Center

Nursing Management of Geriatric Patient

- ☑ Geriatric Assessment
- ☑ Fall Risk Assessment

Geriatric Assessment

EVALUATION CRITERIA FOR GERIATRIC ASSESSMENT

Maximum Marks: 25

S. No.	Contents	Maximum marks	Marks obtained
1.	Patient's history	05	
2.	Physical assessment	10	
3.	Abnormalities detected	05	
4.	Conclusion	05	
	Total	**25**	

Remarks:

Signature of Student   **Signature of Supervisor**

Patient's Identification Data

- Name :
- Age :
- Sex :
- Marital status :
- Hospital registration no. :
- Ward/bed no. :
- Address :
- Tel. no. :
- Religion :
- Education :
- Date of admission :
- Date of discharge :
- Diagnosis :
- Operation :
- Date of operation :
- Name of the doctor :
- Occupation :
- Monthly family income (₹) :
- Nursing alert :
- Sensitivity/allergy/precaution :
- Weight :
- Height :

Informant

Information's relevant or not.

Personal History

- Habits

- Healthy practices

- Diet

- Hobbies

Present Medical History

Past Medical History

Physical Examination Personal Appearance

Scalp

- Color of the hair:

- Any wound or birth markings:

Face and Neck

- Eyes (color, cataract, vision):

- Ear (hearing):

- Nose (running, blocked, deviation):

- Mouth (teeth, odor any abnormality):

- Tongue:

- Throat:

- Distension of neck veins:

Abdomen

- Any distension:

- Auscultation:

- Percussion:

- Bowel and bladder movements:

Extremities

- Musculoskeletal pain:

- Postmenopausal symptoms:

- Any abnormalities seen:

- Movements of joints:

Abnormalities Detected

Suggestion Given

Conclusion

Fall Risk Assessment

▌EVALUATION CRITERIA FOR FALL RISK ASSESSMENT

Maximum Marks: 20

S. No.	Contents	Maximum marks	Marks obtained
1.	Patient's history	05	
2.	Fall risk assessment tool	10	
3.	Conclusion	05	
	Total	**20**	

Remarks:

Signature of Student

Signature of Supervisor

Patient's Identification Data

- Name :
- Age :
- Sex :
- Marital status :
- Hospital registration no. :
- Ward/bed no. :
- Address :
- Tel. no. :
- Religion :
- Education :
- Date of admission :
- Date of discharge :
- Diagnosis :
- Operation :
- Date of operation :
- Name of the doctor :
- Occupation :
- Monthly family income (₹) :
- Nursing alert :
- Sensitivity/allergy/precaution :
- Weight :
- Height :

Informant

Information's relevant or not.

Fall Risk Assessment Tool

Fall risk score calculation: Select the appropriate option in each category. Add all points to calculate fall risk score (if no option is selected, score for category is 0)	Score
Age (single-select)	
◆ 60–69 years (1 point)	
◆ 70–79 years (2 points)	
◆ Greater than or equal to 80 years (3 points)	
Fall history (single-select)	
One fall within 6 months before admission (5 points)	
Elimination, bowel and urine (single-select)	
◆ Incontinence (2 points)	
◆ Urgency or frequency (2 points)	
◆ Urgency/frequency and incontinence (4 points)	
Medications: Includes PCA/opiates, anticonvulsants, antihypertensives, diuretics, hypnotics, laxatives, sedatives, and psychotropics (single-select)	
◆ On 1 high fall risk drug (3 points)	
◆ On 2 or more high fall risk drugs (5 points)	
◆ Sedated procedure within past 24 hours (7 points)	
Patient care equipment: Any equipment that tethers patient (e.g., IV infusion, chest tube, indwelling catheter, SCDs, etc.) (single-select)	
◆ One present (1 point)	
◆ Two present (2 points)	
◆ Three or more present (3 points)	
Mobility (multi-select, choose all that apply and add points together)	
◆ Requires assistance or supervision for mobility, transfer, or ambulation (2 points)	
◆ Unsteady gait (2 points)	
◆ Visual or auditory impairment affecting mobility (2 points)	
Cognition (multi-select, choose all that apply and add points together)	
◆ Altered awareness of immediate physical environment (1 point)	
◆ Impulsive (2 points)	
◆ Lack of understanding of one's physical and cognitive limitations (4 points)	
Scoring: 6–13 total points = moderate fall risk, >13 total points = high fall risk	

Conclusion